To my daughter, Arabella. You fill my life with love and joy.
You give me incredible pleasure seeing you grow and thrive.
You inspire me to be a better person.

CONTENTS

Introduction: Eat Optimally for Life

Why is it that we don't always do the things we know are good for us? Most of my weight-loss patients are well informed about nutrition and healthy living. They know, for example, that grilled fish and vegetables are a healthier meal choice than a cheeseburger and fries, but that doesn't always ensure they'll make the healthier choice. Even professional dietitians and doctors who specialize in weight loss sometimes struggle with their weight.

What most people don't know, because the research is so new, is how much our hormones are involved in regulating our appetite, metabolism, cravings, and more. The old joke (or excuse?) is true: It's a hormonal problem. Scientists are learning more every day about how hormones influence your weight.

That doesn't mean you have to let your hormones run wild. By reading this book, you can learn how to regulate them with a balanced meal plan and finally lose those pounds for good.

Our hormone levels surge and recede according to several factors, the first of which is, naturally, the type of food we eat. To beat overeating, it's not enough to eat healthy foods; you have to keep it coming, five times a day. Without this reliable schedule, your brain will send out warning signals of starvation, and you'll end up overeating the unhealthy foods that you crave.

This sets up a vicious cycle of hormone disruption. In part two of this book, you'll come to understand which of your hormones is acting out, and how to bring it back in line so you can lose weight and keep it off for life.

GIVE YOURSELF A BREAK

Our hormones are also affected by a human gene pool that has survived famines by conserving fat and hasn't had time to adjust to plentiful food (and fast and fake food). Scientists are also just beginning to learn about the dramatic effect that environmental toxins, such as the bisphenol A (BPA) found in many plastics, have in directing our fat cells to multiply.

If that isn't enough to take yourself off the hook, consider that in recent years, the number of obese American adults has increased by more than 70 percent. Many other countries are experiencing spikes as part of a global obesity epidemic. There is more going on here than your lack of willpower.

In this book, I will show you how to protect and control your hormones by eating wholesome and satisfying meals and snacks. Based on my work with thousands of weight-loss patients, I have developed a BON! Eating Plan that will provide you with the foundation for a lifetime of healthy eating. I encourage you to experiment with new foods, but also recognize that if you learn to cook a few basic dishes, including comfort foods, you'll be more likely to stick to the plan. Look for delicious fundamental recipes in chapter 2.

PUSH THE RESTART BUTTON NOW

I know you want to get right to it, so I've included a list of Action Items at the beginning of every chapter. Keep a lookout for Action Items that you can do right away. Changing your habits can be challenging, so it's important to take it one step at a time. Throughout the book, I'll suggest step-by-step ways for you to add new healthy foods and behaviors into your life.

You don't need to follow every Action Item and shouldn't feel overwhelmed. I want you to read this book thinking about how you can add these healthy behaviors to your life, slowly creating new habits. The longer you practice new healthy behaviors, the more they will become second nature and part of your everyday routine.

My goal for this book is to help you achieve what you already know you should do. Armed with the knowledge that your overeating is largely due to hormonal dysfunction, you can do something about it. By following my plan, you can focus on continuous improvement, one step at a time, to regulate your hormone levels and achieve an ideal weight without ever being hungry again.

—Scott Isaacs, M.D.

PART ONE:
Beat Overeating with My Daily Eating Plan

CHAPTER

1

Prepare to Beat Overeating

Many of my patients have been extremely successful in most aspects of their life, except their weight. They may be a corporate CEO, a judge, or a principal of a school; they may have won awards, honors, and recognitions; the one thing that had evaded them was a healthy weight.

As I have told them, I am telling you now that you can be successful losing weight and keep it off forever. Even if you have failed before, there is still hope for you. The key isn't just what you eat and how much you exercise, but understanding how your hormones are involved in dictating your behaviors and the growth of fat cells.

When scientists discovered the hormone leptin in 1994, the door was opened to one of the most important areas of medical research today. We now know about dozens of hunger hormones that influence your appetite, cravings, metabolism, and body weight. *Beat Overeating Now!* (BON!) will help you bring your hunger hormones back under control to lose weight fast and forever.

Outsmart Your Hunger Hormones

Most overweight people feel hopeless and doomed to be overweight forever, especially when studies show that 98 percent of people who lose weight gain it back. As I tell my patients, you don't need to be in the 98 percent. You can be

actionplan

Beat Overeating

- *Get started now.*
- *Use a "to-do" approach.*
- *Understand what you are up against.*
- *Set realistic goals.*
- *Anticipate and plan.*
- *Buy healthy foods.*
- *Eat the right amount of food and balance of nutrients.*

part of the elite 2 percent who finally learn what and when to eat to outsmart their hunger hormones. It's not hard to do. This book will show you how to beat overeating and lose weight permanently.

As an endocrinologist, I've treated thousands of people who are trying to lose weight by learning about their hormones. I've observed that the successful 2 percent do things differently than other "dieters." For one thing, they never let themselves get hungry, but eat five times a day. I reveal the eating and lifestyle behaviors of my successful patients in Action Plans for each chapter. You don't have to do them all, but the more healthy behaviors you adopt, the more weight you'll lose.

Get Started Right Now

The time to start losing weight is now. Don't wait a minute longer. All you need to do is add one healthy behavior. As you read this book, look for Action Items that you can do immediately to start forming new habits as soon as possible. There is no reason to wait until you've finished reading the whole book.

Permanent weight loss requires a long-term effort to make sustainable lifestyle changes. But you don't need to do everything all at once. Right now, take the first step. Get started with an easily attainable goal: Eat one piece of fruit or go for a walk today. Build on your success by eating more healthy foods and exercising more tomorrow. If you are waiting for permission to be healthy, I am giving you that permission. All you need to do is to get started.

TAKE A WATER BREAK

Here's something healthy you can do right now: Stop reading this book and go have a glass of water. As you'll read in chapter 7, drinking enough water every day is an important step to staying hydrated, decreasing appetite, keeping your metabolism humming, and balancing hormones. It's a necessary step to beating overeating.

Big changes come with small steps, so I've also included a series of Step by Step sidebars that suggest ways to do things differently.

It's important to make changes now to improve your health—if not for you, for your children and loved ones. As a parent, spouse, sibling, or friend, you have an obligation to be a healthy role model. We hope to live a long life, watching children grow into healthy adults. No one wants to realize too late that they have crippled their children with eating habits that prohibit a happy, healthy life.

Use a "To-do" Approach

Your first step on this program is to start adding healthy foods and behaviors. You don't have to be perfect to be successful. I recommend adding healthy behaviors one by one, starting with the Action Items that you can do right now. Once you start a new healthy behavior, keep doing this until it becomes a habit and part of your regular routine. Then add another Action Item. The more you do, the better.

Focus on continuous self-improvement by adding healthy behaviors, step by step. Sometimes, these new behaviors will feel uncomfortable or unnatural. For example, it may be very difficult to begin exercising every morning before you go to work. Learn to accept the uncomfortable feeling as part of your growth and change. But don't push it so much that a new behavior backfires and you revolt. Perhaps you could begin by exercising before work once a week. The habit might grow into something you enjoy and love to do.

Remember that change is difficult at first but necessary to reach your goals. Push yourself enough to keep your weight moving in the right direction, but don't overdo it to the point where you feel restricted and unsatisfied. Keep a positive frame of mind by concentrating on adding healthy behaviors, not restricting unhealthy ones. Small steps make changes feel less overwhelming.

FOCUS ON ADDING HEALTHY BEHAVIORS

For losing weight, adding more healthy behaviors is more effective than trying to eliminate unhealthy behaviors.

According to the North American Association for the Study of Obesity, dieters who focused on increasing their consumption of healthy foods lost 40 percent more weight in six months than those who relied on reducing portion sizes and limiting fat intake. Other studies, including one from Utrecht University in The Netherlands, have shown that taking a restrictive, "not to-do" approach is ineffective and can have a rebound effect that results in weight gain!

Be Different in a Good Way

Although the majority of Americans are overweight, research shows that a minority of its citizens are actively trying to lose weight. Remember, to be part of the elite 2 percent, you need to do things differently than most others. If you start right now, that makes you one of those people actively trying to lose weight.

Five Don'ts

Focusing on what *to do* is the best approach to losing weight, but there are a handful of don'ts:

DON'T:

- Deprive yourself of calories and nutrients.
- Avoid delicious and satisfying foods.
- Eat a lot of processed foods or fake foods.
- Eat a lot of unhealthy foods such as fast food, candy, cookies, and cakes.
- Give up.

There are so many things you shouldn't do that focusing on the negatives can be overwhelming. Taking a "to-do" approach will allow you to slowly add healthy behaviors, making consistent small changes that you can build on. The key is not to move backward, but ever onward with established healthy habits, and then adding in more steps.

Be Done with Diets; Eat for Life

Diets don't work. Just thinking about going on another diet can be depressing. Diets are restrictive and punitive. Diets don't give you a plan for eating for the rest of your life. Diets usually feature foods that you don't like very much and that aren't very satisfying.

Most people stick it out on a diet so they can achieve a weight-loss goal, but are miserable while they are doing it. Being on a diet implies that one day you will go off the diet. When this happens, weight is quickly regained.

I want you to think of the BON! Eating Plan as a guide for eating daily for the rest of your life, not something that you go on or off. This will help you make healthy choices without forcing you into a rigid diet.

Understand What You Are Up Against

Obesity is one of the greatest health challenges our planet has ever faced. According to the World Health Organization, there are more than 1 billion overweight and 300 million obese adults in the world. In the past few years, the number of obese adults in the United States has increased by 74 percent to more than one 120 million.

In the 1980s, Americans started gaining weight, and by the 1990s, experts agreed that obesity rates had reached "epidemic" proportions. More than 70 percent of Americans are now obese or overweight, and the numbers continue to increase. Many other countries are also experiencing an epidemic of obesity. This is a worldwide problem. You are a victim of this epidemic.

"THRIFTY" GENES ARE THE CULPRITS

Experts who study the obesity epidemic tell us that the cause lies in our genes. You may have heard about this "thrifty gene" hypothesis, which notes that our bodies are genetically programmed to gain weight.

Until very recently in the history of humankind, starvation was a major cause of death. As the genetic "survival of the fittest" game went on over millennia, this theory goes, the people who survived and spawned offspring were the ones with thrifty genes who conserved body fat and were prone to weight gain. The people with fast metabolisms died in famines.

Our modern-day environment does not bode well for the thrifty genes of our ancestors. Now that food is plentiful, there is no benefit to having them, but the genetic pool has not had time to change. We are still living on the genetic selections made by environmental pressures from thousands of years ago.

MEET YOUR HUNGER HORMONES

Your thrifty genes control hormones that boost your appetite and make you crave food. These hunger hormones are made by the organs involved in making you fat: fat cells, the stomach, intestines, pancreas, and brain. Hunger hormones have various effects on your appetite, satiety (ability to feel full and satisfied), and cravings. They slow your metabolism and make you gain weight.

The good news is that although you can't change your genes, there is a lot you can do to get your hunger hormones to work with you instead of against you.

Why Knowledge Will Help You Beat Overeating

Researchers from the University of Marburg in Germany found that knowledge helps people lose weight because they gain insight about their bodies and what they can do to tip the scales in their favor.

Knowledge about the genetics of obesity also takes you off the hook. Instead of feeling guilty, you need to know how your body works. Thrifty genes tell your hunger hormones to overeat. But you can fool your hunger hormones. Throughout this book, I'll give you better insight into your body so you can lose weight and keep it off permanently.

DON'T BLAME YOURSELF

If you are overweight or obese, you are part of a worldwide epidemic. It is not your fault. Your genes and hormones are making you fat.

Researchers say people who blame themselves for being overweight are rarely successful with a weight-loss program. Their shame, guilt, and negative self-image lead to an inability to cope with stress such as changing one's behavior. If you need to place blame, blame your genes and hormones.

Acknowledge that you are capable of making changes and achieving your goals. You can be the solution. You can overcome your hormones and genetics to beat overeating.

Set Realistic Goals

Eating on a schedule is a very important part of the BON! Eating Plan. To accomplish this, you will have to plan your meals and snacks in advance. Don't leave anything to chance. Write down your menu and display it so you can see what you will eat and when. Be as specific as possible, but be realistic.

Understand that goals should not be "all or nothing." Try to focus on small improvements instead of being perfect. Overloading yourself with too much at once can make you burn out.

Check up on yourself. Assess and reassess your progress, adjusting goals when necessary. Be persistent and determined to achieve your goals, especially when there are challenges.

STEP BY STEP

Ways to Keep Your Goals

- Keep a food journal with a plan for what and when you are going to eat.
- Make a plan for the short term (one day, or even one hour at a time).
- Focus on long-term success by adding sustainable behaviors.
- Commit to your goals and following your plan.
- Think about your goals every day and find the time to act on them.
- Avoid situations that will tempt you to deviate from your goals.

Determine Your Ideal Body Weight

The best way to determine your ideal body weight is by using the Body Mass Index (BMI). This calculation presents a numerical value based on the ratio of your height and weight. The BMI is in metrics—kilograms per meters squared. There are many BMI calculators on the Internet. All you need to know is your height and weight. Or you can use this simple formula:

BMI = (weight in pounds) x 703 / [(height in inches) x (height in inches)]

For example, if you weigh 180 pounds and you are 5 foot 6 inches, BMI = (180 x 703) / (66 x 66) = 29 kg/m^2

BMI (kg/m^2)	Weight category
<18.4	Underweight
18.5–24.9	Normal weight
25–29.9	Overweight
30–34.9	Class I obesity
35–39.9	Class II obesity
40–59.9	Class III obesity
>60	"Extreme" obesity

Your long-term goal should be a normal BMI of 20 to 25 kg/m^2, which is a healthy weight for most people.

You can have a normal BMI and still be unhealthy. If you are out of shape and have flabby muscles and a high percentage of body fat, you may be what is known as "normal weight metabolically obese."

On the other hand, if you have a lot of muscle and a very low body fat percentage, a BMI that is slightly higher than 25 kg/m^2 may be a healthy weight for you.

SETTING A WEIGHT-LOSS GOAL

Your long-term goal is to have a normal body weight, but you should have a realistic short-term goal as well. A reasonable short-term goal is to lose 5 to 10 percent of your body weight. If you weigh 200 pounds (91 kg), concentrate on losing the first 20 pounds (9 kg), or 10 percent, as your short-term goal.

Doctors consider a 5 to 10 percent weight loss to be medically significant because it can have a beneficial impact on weight-related medical problems, such as blood pressure and diabetes control.

Achieve Goals Unrelated to Weight

Achieving a normal body weight is not the only goal you should have. You can set other goals that are specific to your health, such as controlling diabetes, blood pressure, or high cholesterol—or reducing or discontinuing medications.

You could have a specific fitness goal, such as running a 10K or a marathon, or swimming a mile. If you're just starting an exercise program, exercising once a week to exercising every day is a reasonable goal.

You might also have goals for other aspects of your health and appearance, such as understanding basic nutrition and portion sizes, getting good quality sleep, ridding the toxins from your life, or fitting into a certain size of clothes. Your goals should be customized to meet your specific needs and reevaluated as time goes on.

The Importance of Planning Ahead

Successful long-term weight loss requires that you do a lot of planning. The more you plan and prepare for, the more likely you'll stick to it and the greater your odds of success. You will need to plan your meals and snacks. Don't go out for the day without a defined plan about what you are going to eat that day and how you are going to exercise. Researchers at the University of Sydney in Australia found that planned healthy behaviors, such as planning to eat breakfast or planning to exercise, can be useful for translating your intentions into action.

Continue to learn about nutrition and a healthy lifestyle. Determine exactly what it will take (what, when, how) to meet your goals each day. Look for opportunities to meet them instead of excuses not to. What challenges lie ahead? Plan for unexpected changes in the day. For example, if you normally exercise outside, have a contingency plan in case the weather is bad.

Have a plan for getting started on your new healthy program and a plan to improve as you go along. Plan to continue the healthy behaviors for the long run to keep the weight off.

DON'T OVEREAT IN ANTICIPATION OF GOING ON A DIET

A study from the University of Toronto found that just the anticipation of going on a diet triggered overeating and caused people to gain weight. Remember, your plan is to add healthy behaviors to your life. You are not going on a diet and need never do that again.

CONTROL YOUR ENVIRONMENT

Make an effort to have a lot of healthy food available and keep unhealthy foods out of your home and out of sight. Keep your home clean and organized. People who do a good job of maintaining a healthy, clean, and organized home tend to have less stress and an easier time losing weight.

PREVENT A RELAPSE

Losing weight is hard enough, but keeping it off is even more difficult. Anticipate that maintaining weight loss will be a challenge. You will need to continue to work on developing new healthy behaviors even after you've lost weight.

ENLIST SOCIAL SUPPORT

Studies have shown that you'll be more successful losing weight if you have the support of your family and friends. Tell everyone you know about your goals. See chapter 11 for more information on this important topic.

Focus Goals on Behaviors, Not Weight

A Swiss study found that overweight participants in a weight-loss program were more successful if health-related goals were directed toward the positive behaviors that result in weight loss rather than the weight itself.

Anticipate Regret to Help You Act on Your Intentions

If you plan on doing something unhealthy—or not doing something healthy—think long and hard about how that will make you feel. For example, if you eat an unhealthy food or skip a workout, you're likely to regret it.

Think about how disappointed you'll be in yourself if you don't achieve your goal. Studies have shown that anticipating the regret you'll have by not doing something you were supposed to do is a powerful cue to help you stay on track to accomplish your health goals.

Beat Overeating Now! Shopping List

FRESH FRUITS AND VEGETABLES

(Purchase enough to have 35 to 70 servings per week.)

Apples	Celery	Onions
Artichokes	Cherries	Oranges
Asparagus	Cucumber	Peaches
Bananas	Eggplant	Pears
Beets	Grapefruit	Pineapple
Bell peppers	Grapes	Plums
Blueberries	Green beans	Raspberries
Broccoli	Honeydew melon	Spinach
Brussels sprouts	Lemons	Strawberries
Cabbage	Lettuce	Tomatoes
Cantaloupe	Mango	Watermelon
Carrots	Mushrooms	Yellow squash
Cauliflower	Okra	Zucchini

Frozen fruits and vegetables can be substituted for fresh. Canned vegetables and fruits are okay if they're stored in BPA-free cans and without added sugar. Low-sodium canned vegetables are better than the regular sodium versions. Do not buy dried fruit.

GRAINS AND STARCHES

Corn	Quinoa
Healthy breakfast cereals	Steel-cut oats (not instant)
Lentils	Sweet potatoes
Peas	Whole-grain bread
Potatoes	Wild rice

Beat Overeating Now! Shopping List (cont.)

SPICES AND CONDIMENTS

Basil	Garlic	Oregano
Black pepper	Ginger	Rosemary
Chili powder	Hot sauce	Sugar-free pudding mix or gelatin powder (to flavor smoothies)
Cinnamon	Mint	Turmeric
Dark chocolate	Mustard	Vinegar

PROTEINS
(Buy organic or hormone-free whenever possible.)

Beans or chickpeas (dried or canned)	Fish	Powdered smoothie mix
Chicken breast	Lean beef	Turkey breast
Eggs	Lentils	

LOW-FAT DAIRY PRODUCTS
(Buy organic or hormone-free whenever possible.)

Fat-free cottage cheese	Greek yogurt	Low-fat mozzarella string cheese
Fat-free sour cream	Low-fat frozen yogurt	Skim milk (small container)
Frozen dessert treats		

BEVERAGES

Coffee	Diet soda water	Tea

Create and Guard a Positive Mind-set

Focus on the positive aspects of your life and your ability to adopt healthy behaviors. Be grateful for all the good things you have in your life. Negative thoughts and self-blame lead to weight gain, according to a recent study of attitudes relating to weight-loss goals. Having a positive outlook helps you feel motivated to adopt better health-related coping skills.

Motivate yourself by creating a positive environment that is conducive for weight loss and makes relapse to poor habits less likely.

Buy Healthy Foods

My successful patients make it a point to keep their kitchens stocked with the food they need to accomplish their goals. Clean out your refrigerator and pantry. Throw away the unhealthy foods and replace them with healthy ones. Where would you rather have all those unhealthy foods—in your body or the garbage can? Throw them away and get a fresh start.

Plan to shop at least once a week so that you can have the fresh foods on hand that you need to follow the BON! Eating Plan. Shop the perimeter of a grocery store, where most of the foods on the BON! Eating Plan are located.

DON'T WORRY ABOUT COUNTING EVERY CALORIE

Knowing about calories, nutrients, and portions is important for losing weight, but it is not the be-all and end-all. Many of my patients are very aware of what they need to do, but still struggle with implementing healthy behaviors. If you focus on the Action Plans in this book, you can lose a lot of weight without counting every calorie.

Most people lose 1 to 2 pounds (0.5 to 1 kg) per week in the weight-loss phase, but this can vary. I always tell my patients that even if you eat exactly the same food and exercise the same amount, your actual weight loss can vary from week to week.

Don't get too caught up in the amount of weight you lose in a day or in a week. Things other than fat, such as water and bowel contents, can affect short-term weight changes and can be misleading. It is better to assess your progress by looking at your four-week weight-loss average.

Eat the Right Amount of Food, with Balanced Nutrients

No matter what you do, you can't change the laws of physics. Weight loss ultimately comes down to the number of calories consumed and burned. It is hard to count calories all the time, but you may need to be more compulsive about knowing the calories in what you eat, especially in the beginning.

As I discuss in chapter 7, it's essential to regulate your hormones by eating balanced meals and balanced calories throughout the day. A balanced meal includes about 40 percent carbohydrates, 30 percent protein, and 30 percent fat. You should spread your calorie intake across breakfast, lunch, an afternoon snack, dinner, and dessert, as I discuss in chapter 2.

A Guide to Weight Loss and Maintenance

Use the chart to determine the number of calories and grams of carbohydrates, protein, and fat you should consume in a day, according to your body weight and gender, and if you are trying to maintain weight or lose weight.

Men (Weight Loss)									
Body weight (pounds)	125-150	150-175	175-200	200-225	225-250	250-275	275-300	300-325	325-350
Calories per day	1100	1200	1400	1600	1800	2000	2200	2400	2600
Carbohydrates (grams per day)	110	120	140	160	180	200	220	240	260
Protein (grams per day)	83	90	105	120	135	150	165	180	195
Fat (grams per day)	37	40	47	53	60	67	73	80	87
Men (Weight Maintenance)									
Body weight (pounds)	125-150	150-175	175-200	200-225	225-250	250-275	275-300	300-325	325-350
Calories per day	1300	1500	1700	1900	2100	2400	2700	3000	3300
Carbohydrates (grams per day)	130	150	170	190	210	240	270	300	330
Protein (grams per day)	98	112	130	145	160	180	205	225	250
Fat (grams per day)	44	50	56	63	70	80	90	100	110

(continued on page 24)

A Guide to Weight Loss and Maintenance *(cont.)*

Women (Weight Loss)									
Body weight (pounds)	125–150	150–175	175–200	200–225	225–250	250–275	275–300	300–325	325–350
Calories per day	1000	1100	1200	1400	1600	1800	2000	2200	2400
Carbohydrates (grams per day)	100	110	120	160	180	200	220	240	260
Protein (grams per day)	75	83	90	120	135	150	165	180	195
Fat (grams per day)	33	37	40	53	60	67	73	80	87
Women (Weight Maintenance)									
Body weight (pounds)	125–150	150–175	175–200	200–225	225–250	250–275	275–300	300–325	325–350
Calories per day	1200	1300	1500	1700	1900	2100	2400	2700	3000
Carbohydrates (grams per day)	120	130	150	170	190	210	240	270	300
Protein (grams per day)	90	97	112	127	142	158	180	202	225
Fat (grams per day)	40	43	50	57	64	70	80	90	100

Eat to Outsmart Your Hunger Hormones

The BON! Eating Plan is simple and wholesome, the way people used to eat before processed foods became the convenient staples of the pantry. After all, it's only natural that our bodies can get all the nutrients we need from foods that grow on Earth. By contrast, eating nutrient-poor fake food upsets your natural hormone balance and makes your body crave more food, which results in overeating. Fake foods increase your appetite and cravings because your body is still searching for nutrients and because of the addictive additives in fake food.

Eat Right to Fight Hunger and Cravings

Eating real food, whether it's a small pad of butter instead of margarine or crumpled bacon instead of bacon bits, will leave you far more satisfied for longer periods of time. The BON! Eating Plan is the opposite of a diet, which limits your intake of specific foods and leaves you feeling hungry and deprived. Instead, it's an eating plan that will get your hormones back on track and the scale pointing toward your ideal weight. You'll feast on delicious foods at breakfast, lunch, afternoon snack, dinner, and dessert. Feel free to overeat the right foods—you need never be hungry again!

*action*plan

Eat Well for Life

- *Balance your carbs, fat, and protein at every meal.*
- *Aim for five servings of vegetables and five servings of fruits every day.*
- *Eat a big breakfast with protein.*
- *Eat a healthy balanced lunch.*
- *Eat an afternoon snack with protein.*
- *Eat healthy comfort foods at dinner.*
- *Eat a sweet, slow-carbohydrate dessert.*
- *Learn to make a few simple healthy dishes for which you can change the ingredients to create variety.*

Stick to the Routine

If an acronym like BLADD (for Breakfast, Lunch, Afternoon snack, Dinner, and Dessert) helps you stick to the plan, terrific. Whatever works. To beat overeating, you need to eat on this schedule and not skip any meals or snacks. You might not feel hungry enough to eat small meals at these times, but you need to eat all five meals anyway. This helps balance your hormones and prevents hunger later in the day, when you are more likely to overeat.

When Cravings Strike, Chew Gum

A study from England found that chewing gum can help suppress appetite and reduce cravings for high-calorie snacks for about forty-five minutes.

Balance Your Macronutrients

Macronutrients are the key nutritional components of food: carbohydrates, protein, and fat. A healthy, balanced diet contains 40 percent carbohydrates, 30 percent protein, and 30 percent fat.

Macronutrients can be "healthy" or "unhealthy." Healthy carbohydrates, such as vegetables, fruits, whole grains, and low-fat dairy products, help you lose weight because of their effect on insulin (see chapter 5), gut hormones (see chapter 6), and leptin (see chapter 7). Healthy proteins, including meats and fish, are without a lot of fat. It is also important to consume the right amount of healthy fat (see chapter 7).

Vegetables and Fruits Are Fundamental to the Plan

No matter what, you need to make sure you eat enough vegetables and fruits every day. Your goal is to eat a minimum of five servings each of vegetables and fruits. There is no limit. You can eat as many vegetables and fruits as you want.

The best strategy is to substitute vegetables and fruits for higher calorie foods. As I discuss in chapter 3, you should "eat the rainbow" by choosing a variety of colors of vegetables and fruits, which flood the body with beneficial vitamins and minerals and keep appetite low.

HOW TO MEASURE SERVINGS

It is important to understand what constitutes a serving size. In general, a serving of vegetables or fruit is 1 cup. The actual serving size varies depending on how large the pieces are. For example, larger items have air between the pieces, but when chopped are more compact, so a smaller amount can make up a serving. Cooking sometimes makes a vegetable smaller, so cooked vegetables may have a smaller serving size. Because you should always focus on eating more vegetables and fruits, not less, if there is any doubt as to what constitutes a serving, just round up and err on the side of eating more vegetables and fruits.

Step by Step: What's in a Serving?

Fruits	1 cup
Vegetables (raw)	1 cup
Vegetables (cooked)	½ to 1 cup
Salad greens	2 cups

MORE SPECIFIC VEGETABLE SERVINGS

Bean sprouts (cooked)	1 cup (50 g)
Bell pepper (any color)	1 large
Broccoli (chopped, cooked)	¾ cup (70 g)
Broccoli (florets, cooked)	1 cup (70 g)
Broccoli	Three 5-inch (13 cm) spears
Cabbage (chopped, cooked)	¾ cup (113 g)
Carrots (baby)	1 cup (80 g)
Carrots	2 medium
Cauliflower (chopped, cooked)	¾ cup (75 g)
Cauliflower (florets, cooked)	1 cup (75 g)

Celery	3 medium stalks
Corn	1 large ear
Mushrooms (chopped, cooked)	½ cup (75 g)
Mushrooms (chopped, raw)	1 cup (75 g)
Potato (white or sweet)	One 2½-inch (6.4 cm) whole
Spinach (chopped, cooked)	½ cup (15 g)
Tomato	1 large

MORE SPECIFIC FRUIT SERVINGS

Apple	1 small or ½ large
Banana	1 large
Grapefruit	One 4-inch (10 cm) (medium)
Grapes	30
Orange	One 3½-inch (9 cm) (medium)
Peach	One 2½-inch (6.4 cm) (large)
Pear	1 medium
Plum	3 medium or 2 large
Strawberries	10 to 12 medium

Time Well Spent in the Kitchen

The time you spend preparing and eating your breakfast is an investment in your health and well-being. When you eat breakfast, you have more energy and your brain works better, making you more productive all day.

ALWAYS ADD EXTRA VEGETABLES

You will never go wrong adding extra vegetables. Think of it this way: The more vegetables you eat, the more weight you will lose. At meals, fill up your plate with vegetables. Add a salad. Snack on raw vegetables. Order a side order of extra veggies at a restaurant. You can even hide the vegetables. Researchers at Penn State found that hiding vegetables in food, perhaps by adding them to a spaghetti sauce, helps people consume more of them, leading to weight loss. Jessica Seinfeld's book *Deceptively Delicious* embraces this idea with delicious recipes that contain lots of hidden vegetables and fruits.

Use a Straw

Drink your smoothie through a straw to slow down your consumption, allowing your gut hormones to start working to suppress your appetite.

Smooth and Easy

INGREDIENTS

6 to 8 ounces (175 to 235 ml) water

1 to 2 cups (250 to 500 g) frozen fruit (strawberries, blueberries, raspberries, blackberries, cherries, pineapple, peaches, mangoes, etc.)

2 scoops of protein powder or low-calorie shake mix, or 1 cup (230 g) fat-free vanilla yogurt or ¾ cup (175 g) Greek yogurt

4 to 6 ice cubes

DIRECTIONS

Add water and half of the fruit to the blender and blend on low. Continue adding fruit until blended. Next, add protein powder or yogurt and continue blending on low. Blend in a few ice cubes until the desired consistency is achieved. Adding in a little more water and ice will also whip in more air, adding volume to the smoothie, which makes you feel fuller.

FLAVORINGS

Try different combinations of fruits and add flavorings to your smoothies so you don't get bored having the same ones all the time. You also can try adding some fresh spinach or some cooked squash as a way of getting in extra vegetables. As I discuss in chapter 5, you should limit artificial sweeteners, but you can have a small amount in a smoothie.

- Extracts (vanilla, peppermint, almond, coconut, etc.)
- Cocoa (unsweetened)
- Sugar-free pudding mix (1 teaspoon max per smoothie)
- Sugar-free gelatin powder (1 teaspoon max per smoothie)
- Sugar-free syrups
- PB2 peanut butter powder
- Coffee or espresso
- Tea or green tea
- Cinnamon
- Nutmeg

Protein Is Essential to the Daily Eating Plan

Of the three macronutrients—carbohydrates, protein, and fat—protein is by far the most satisfying. This is why it is such an important component of a healthy diet. You might think that high-fat foods would be more satisfying, but studies have shown that protein packs a more powerful punch, reducing appetite and cravings for a longer period of time.

Protein takes a long time to chew, which slows down eating, allowing the gut hormones to send the "I'm full" signal to your brain. Throughout this chapter, I often refer to "protein" in various meals and recipes. You can substitute different types of protein in your meals to increase your variety of healthy foods. Always strive to choose the lowest-fat options for proteins (see chapter 7).

Become a Master Smoothie Maker

I recommend that you become an expert at making shakes and smoothies. A smoothie is a shake with fruit blended in. Smoothies are better than shakes because they allow you to consume more fruits (and vegetables) and increase the amount of fiber and nutrients you consume. Countless studies reveal the weight-loss benefits of shakes and smoothies. Smoothies are extremely filling because of their effect on gut hormones such as ghrelin and PYY (see chapter 6).

Low-calorie weight-loss shake powders are available at grocery stores, health food stores, and from a variety of Internet retailers. Milk- and soy-based weight-loss shake powders are available. Be aware that consuming too much soy can cause thyroid and sex hormone dysfunction (see chapter 5).

It's True: Breakfast Is the Most Important Meal

You have heard it many times because it's true. You must eat breakfast. According to the National Weight Control Registry, the successful minority of people who have lost weight and kept it off make it a habit to eat breakfast every day. Some people think they can save calories by skipping breakfast, but it ends up backfiring. If you skip breakfast, your ghrelin will surge and your PYY will plummet; your hunger will explode and you will end up overeating all day. When you

What Constitutes Protein?

When I refer to "protein" in a meal or a recipe, it means:

- Chicken breast
- Turkey breast
- Lean beef, pork, or lamb
- Lean ground meat (chicken or turkey breast, beef, pork, lamb)
- Fish
- Shrimp, scallops, lobster, or crab
- Bison, elk, or venison
- Tofu
- Chopped, hard-boiled eggs (mostly whites)
- Vegetable protein (beans, chickpeas, soy, lentils)

Build Up to a Big Breakfast

An effective technique is to start off slow. Eat a very small breakfast every day for a week or two. Gradually increase the amount of food you eat for breakfast until you are able to eat a big breakfast.

eat breakfast, your metabolism is revved up because your body doesn't think it is starving. Eating breakfast controls your appetite for the entire day.

Many of my patients tell me that they don't eat breakfast because they don't feel hungry in the morning. It may not be surprising to know that people who overeat often skip breakfast. Eating breakfast doesn't always feel natural, even for people who do not overeat. It is not always easy to do.

It may be a challenge, but this is something you can do—and remember, the more you do, the more you will beat overeating and lose weight. Even if you don't feel hungry, eat breakfast anyway. With time, your body will become accustomed to getting calories in the morning. Your food intake will shift so that you are eating more calories earlier in the day and less food in the afternoon and evening. After a few days, you will start feeling hungrier at breakfast. Your body will start craving breakfast, which is a good thing.

HIGH-CARB BREAKFASTS LEAD TO CRAVINGS

High-carbohydrate breakfasts have been shown in studies to boost appetite. In chapter 5, I talk about how eating a high-carbohydrate, low-protein breakfast makes your blood sugar and insulin levels surge, causing cravings for sugars or starchy foods later in the day. Eating protein at breakfast, on the other hand, reduces appetite and cravings, and helps you stick with the eating plan all day long.

Step by Step: Feed Your Hormones at Breakfast

Eating a BON! breakfast is one of the most important things you can do to feel less hungry as you stop overeating. As you read this book, you will come to understand how all your hormones need a big high-protein breakfast to work at their optimal levels.

Aim to eat about 30 percent of your daily calories at breakfast. The meal should contain 30 to 40 percent of high-quality protein, such as three or four egg whites and 2 ounces (55 g) of lean turkey sausage, which translates to about 30 grams of protein for a 150-pound person.

EGGS, A BOUNTY OF PROTEIN

Eggs are one of the easiest ways to get protein at breakfast. Eggs, especially egg whites, are a very healthy and satisfying food. There are 6 to 7 grams (depending on the size of the egg) of high-quality protein and 2 grams of fat (all saturated fat) in an egg. All the protein is in the egg white, and all the fat is in the yolk. Egg whites are considered a "free food," meaning you can eat as much as you want. Egg yolks have unhealthy fat. You don't have to avoid every egg yolk, but eat fewer yolks and more whites. If you want to eat a few egg yolks, keep two yolks and discard the other ten for every dozen eggs you eat.

The protein in eggs helps you to feel full for a long time and gives you energy. One study showed that eggs for breakfast prevents hunger, increases satiety, and reduces calorie intake during the day. Another study showed that eggs are better than a bagel at suppressing ghrelin, and results in less blood sugar and insulin swings.

Variety Increases Appetite for Breakfast

Since variety increases appetite, try to increase the variety of your breakfast repertoire. Most people don't vary their breakfasts very much, eating the same thing on most days. Try new breakfasts and explore items you may have never eaten for breakfast.

Fast, Fluffy Eggs

It's quick and easy to scramble a lot of egg whites with a few of the yolks, or boil the eggs and discard most of the cooked yolks. Here are some ideas to spice up the dish:

- Add vegetables to an omelet, quiche, or frittata.
- Scramble in pieces of lean protein such as ham, turkey, or chicken.
- Try mixing in smoked salmon, crab, shrimp, scallops, or lobster.
- Add a small amount of low-fat cheese.
- Make a veggie scramble with chopped tomato, mushrooms, peppers, asparagus, or onions.
- Whisk 1 to 2 teaspoons of chopped herbs, such as basil, oregano, or parsley, into the eggs before cooking to add extra flavor.
- Use a tiny amount of olive oil* to cook.
- Eggs cook quickly, so use low to medium heat.

*For better cooking, use regular olive oil, not extra virgin (which is better for salad dressing and noncooked foods).

A Morning Snack Is Optional

You can have an optional morning snack to help control hunger and cravings later in the day. One of the best morning snacks is a cup of vegetables, even if you think of it as a supplement. Try microwaved florets of broccoli with pepper to wake up your mouth, or douse mixed vegetables with garlic. See chapter 3 for more information. Simple fruits such as an apple or banana are easy to grab on the run.

TASTY EGG-FREE BREAKFASTS

Some of my patients tell me they don't want to eat eggs every day for breakfast. You don't need to eat eggs to get your protein for breakfast. Some of my patients have found that a healthy sandwich is an extremely satisfying breakfast.

NON-EGG BREAKFASTS HIGH IN PROTEIN

- High-protein breakfast cereal (read the label) with skim milk
- Steel-cut oatmeal with fruit
- Greek yogurt with fruit and chopped nuts
- Fat-free cottage cheese with fruit
- Smoothie
- Low-fat turkey sausage or chicken sausage with fruit
- Any protein (chicken breast, fish, beef, etc.) with fruit
- Sandwich with protein made with whole-grain bread
- Smoked salmon, fat-free cream cheese, tomato, and onion on whole-grain toast

CHOOSE LOW-FAT DAIRY FOR WEIGHT LOSS

Low-fat dairy products are great for weight loss because they are very filling and don't have a lot of calories. They have a low glycemic index, and are high in protein. In addition, dairy products are high in calcium (you need 1200 to 1500 mg daily). Research has shown that getting enough calcium improves weight loss.

Plan Ahead for a Healthy Lunch

The key to a healthy lunch is planning. For many people, lunch can be the biggest problem meal of the day. Many people eat fast food or at restaurants for lunch because they have nothing else to eat. Some of my patients skip lunch altogether, then snack on high-calorie foods in the middle of the afternoon and still feel ravenous at supper. Eating a healthy lunch gives you extra energy to prevent those typical afternoon lows many people experience. It also helps prevent evening and nighttime hunger and cravings, a time when many people tend to overeat.

A healthy lunch takes extra effort in preparation. Make it a habit to pack a healthy lunch and bring it to work with you. Packing your lunch is another "to-do" behavior you can start adding into your daily routine right now.

BE SURE TO FILL UP AT LUNCHTIME

Your lunch should contain a lot of vegetables and at least 4 ounces (115 g) of lean protein. Some of my patients have told me that a salad with chopped chicken is an extremely satisfying lunch, while others say that a hot lunch with a protein and vegetables helps them feel full for the rest of the day.

Frozen entrées are an easy option and can be very satisfying when combined with extra frozen vegetables. If you have a freezer at work, keep a few of these on hand at all times. Vegetables are ideal at lunch because they are heavy and filling. Vegetables contain a lot of fiber, which swells in the stomach, having a beneficial effect on your hunger hormones.

STEP BY STEP

Ways to Add Variety to Lunch

- Combine a big salad of veggies, crushed nuts, and protein (chicken, salmon, shrimp, lean steak, etc.).
- Choose grilled protein (fish, chicken, beef, etc.) with a sweet potato or grain and a double portion of vegetables.
- Make a sandwich with lean meat, lettuce, tomato, low-fat cheese, and mustard on whole-grain high-fiber bread.
- Heat up a hearty soup.
- Bake a potato with the skin on and top it with low-fat turkey chili.
- Cook whole-wheat pasta with tomato sauce, vegetables, and protein.
- Try an omelet, quiche, or scrambled eggs.
- Eat leftovers from your healthy dinner the night before.

Use Restaurant Meals as Rewards

Most restaurants don't have great low-calorie options, even if they claim to. Even though there may be healthy items on the menu, restaurants are designed to make you feel hungry. Staying on track with the BON! Eating Plan can be a challenge when you eat in a lot of restaurants. I recommend eating in restaurants on special occasions or as a reward for doing well on this plan. If you have to eat in a restaurant for business or a social event, follow my advice in chapter 10 to decrease blatantly unhealthy foods and appetite-stimulating foods and increase the healthy foods you eat.

Garnish Your Dish

Make your food look delicious with edible garnishes. This helps suppress ghrelin levels and makes you feel more satisfied. See chapter 6 for ideas.

USE AS MANY CONDIMENTS AS YOU WANT

The BON! Eating Plan encourages you to add a lot of condiments, herbs, and spices for flavor and variety. Condiments are considered a free food and make healthy foods delicious.

CONDIMENTS

- Beef, chicken, or vegetable broth
- Black pepper
- Cayenne pepper
- Extracts (vanilla, mint, etc.)
- Fat-free sour cream
- Herbs (oregano, dill, etc.)
- Horseradish
- Hot sauce
- Lemon or lime juice
- Mustard
- Salad dressing (fat-free, low calorie)
- Salsa
- Soy sauce (low sodium)
- Spices
- Vinegar (balsamic, red wine, rice, apple cider, flavored)
- Worcestershire sauce

The All-important Afternoon Snack

The afternoon snack is critical for maintaining blood sugar levels and keeping ghrelin low and PYY high at a time when hunger tends to surge. Most people go five to six hours between lunch and supper. This is too long to fast without fueling your body. You need to eat this snack before you feel hungry. Your afternoon should include at least 10 grams of protein. High-volume and high-fiber snacks are also good at this time of the day to prevent you from overeating at dinner.

Fruits and vegetables are an excellent snack in the afternoon when combined with some protein. It is necessary to plan your snack in advance so you have it ready to eat at the right time. In chapter 6, I discuss the afternoon snack in more detail and give you some ideas for healthy afternoon snacks that have a lot of protein, such as a hard-boiled egg, protein shake, or pieces of cooked, cut-up chicken breast.

Stay Away from "Snack" Foods

Snack foods are high in calories, unhealthy carbohydrates, trans fats, chemicals, and preservatives. Instead of eating traditional snack foods, eat healthy snacks, such as cut-up pieces of cooked chicken or homemade beef jerky.

Healthy Homemade Jerky

Jerky is an excellent snack because it is pure protein. When you make it yourself, you can be sure it is low in fat and chemicals. Commercially made processed meat jerky is not always a good substitute because it contains a lot of salt and chemicals.

INGREDIENTS

1 pound (455 g) lean meat (beef* is preferred, but chicken, turkey, or salmon can also be used)

½ to 1 cup (120 to 235 ml) any type of sauce or marinade or hot sauce, or ½ cup (120 ml) light soy sauce, ¼ cup (60 g) brown sugar, salt, hot pepper flakes, and ground black pepper. (Explore different recipes!)

*flank steak, top sirloin, bottom round steak, eye of round steak, sirloin tip side steak, or tenderloin

DIRECTIONS

Freeze the meat for 20 to 30 minutes (10 minutes for salmon). Slice the meat into ⅛-inch (3 mm) strips and remove any visible fat. Place meat in container and cover with your sauce of choice. Marinate, covered, in the refrigerator for twelve to twenty-four hours.

Preheat oven to 150°F (65°C). Place strips of meat on a wire rack over a foil-lined cookie sheet. Cook for six to ten hours, testing at six hours, and then check hourly. The jerky is finished when it appears firm and dry and cracks when bent, but it should not break in half. Store in a sealed container. Freeze or refrigerate if desired.

Pop Some Edamame

Edamame (soybeans) are a great snack because they are high in protein, crunchy, and packed with nutrients. There are 21 grams of protein and 10 grams of fiber in 1 cup (135 g) of edamame. However, be aware that too much soy can disrupt thyroid function (see chapter 5).

Continue with a Healthy, Balanced Dinner

Many of my patients tell me that they are able to eat healthy all day long, but they overeat at dinner. The best way to eat a healthy dinner is to set yourself up for success by eating healthy foods all day long. Start your day with a big high-protein breakfast, eat a healthy lunch, and have a protein-rich afternoon snack. This reduces hunger so that making a healthy choice at dinner is a doable task.

My advice for dinner is the same as lunch: Eat a balanced meal with healthy protein and lots of vegetables and fruits. Try eating foods you would normally eat for lunch at dinner and vice versa. Make eating a healthy dinner a priority in your life.

COOK DINNER AT HOME

Many of my patients tell me that they frequently eat dinner out because they don't feel like cooking when they come home at the end of the day. If you have this problem, you are not alone—but don't let it be an excuse for eating an unhealthy dinner. You should problem-solve your life to find ways of making a healthy dinner part of your daily routine.

For many people, this means making big batches on the weekend and freezing or keeping meals in the refrigerator for later in the week. Some of my patients have a big healthy salad or soup for dinner because it is quick, easy, and very filling. The key is to take the time to plan to have healthy dinners at home most nights of the week.

COMFORT FOODS DO JUST THAT

Eating healthy comfort foods at dinner helps you satisfy hunger and stick with the BON! Eating Plan for the long run. Comfort foods can help lower stress, which helps keep cortisol levels manageable. Cortisol stimulates appetite and causes fat accumulation and muscle loss. Your body needs to feel satisfied, and eating foods that fit this bill are critical for long-term success. Eating comfort foods on a regular basis helps prevent cravings and keeps you focused on sticking to the plan for the long haul.

DINNERTIME COMFORT FOODS

- Grilled lean beef steak with a baked potato and broccoli
- Grilled fish with zucchini and corn
- Turkey meatloaf with mashed sweet potatoes and spinach
- Chili (vegetarian, turkey, or lean beef)
- Whole-grain pasta with meat sauce or meatballs
- Shepherd's pie made with ground turkey
- Healthy stir-fry with wild rice
- Healthy chicken vegetable soup
- Minestrone soup

STIR-FRY FUNDAMENTALS

If you don't already know how to stir-fry, it's time to learn. A stir-fry helps you get in a lot of vegetables at dinner to help you feel full, and gives you lots of antioxidant micronutrients.

Add vegetables that have a crunch, such as carrots, pea pods, water chestnuts, and celery. Crunchy vegetables help your gut hormones provide feelings of satiety (see chapter 6). You can enjoy your stir-fry with brown or wild rice or whole-grain pasta such as whole-grain soba noodles. The slow-burning carbohydrates from the vegetables and the pasta or rice stabilize blood sugar and provide your body with energy throughout the night, which helps you burn fat while you sleep.

Prebaked Potatoes

Bake a potato for lunch the night before. This saves you time and makes it easier for you to get in a healthy lunch. Heat it up in the microwave at lunch and top it with low-fat turkey chili and a dollop of fat-free sour cream. To get all the fiber and nutrients, make sure you always eat the skin when you eat a potato. Heating, cooling, and reheating a potato changes the chemical structure of the potato starch, reducing the glycemic index. This makes it a slow carbohydrate (see chapter 5).

Getting Used to a New Diet

Studies have shown that after two days on a diet, appetite starts to decrease as your body gets used to foods with fewer calories.

Simple Stir-fry

It's fast and easy to stir-fry with vegetables, protein, and brown rice.

INGREDIENTS

1 tablespoon (15 ml) healthy oil (olive oil, peanut oil, sesame oil, etc.)

1 to 2 cups (100 to 200 g) vegetables, cut into small pieces (asparagus, mushrooms, onions, peppers, broccoli, squash, etc.)

4 to 6 ounces (115 to 170 g) precooked protein (chicken, beef, shrimp, etc.), cut into small pieces

1 to 2 tablespoons (10 to 20 g) crushed garlic (optional)

1 to 2 tablespoons (10 to 20 g) herbs and spices such as garlic, lemon pepper, mint, oregano, or basil (optional)

1 teaspoon crushed hot pepper (optional)

½ teaspoon ginger (optional)

1 tablespoon (15 ml) low-sodium soy sauce (optional)

DIRECTIONS

Heat oil in a wok or skillet on medium-high temperature. Add the vegetables. Cook, stirring often, 3 to 4 minutes. Add protein and stir for 1 to 2 minutes. Add garlic and seasonings and stir for about 1 minute. Add soy sauce. Stir occasionally for 1 to 2 minutes, then serve hot or cool to store.

USE BROTH AS A BASE FOR DISHES AND SOUPS

Chicken or beef broth (or stock) is great to keep around for use in cooking or as a base for soups. Broth is a free food. You can have as much as you want. In chapter 6, I talk about avoiding liquid calories, but broth doesn't have enough calories to cause those problems. In fact, the protein and savory flavor of broth help decrease your appetite.

The best broth is homemade, fat free, low in salt, and free from chemicals. Canned broth can contain BPA and can be high in salt; however, the low-salt versions are okay if you can't make your own. I don't recommend bouillon because it is high in sodium and has chemicals and MSG. Making broth is work, but it is healthier and tastier. Make extra and freeze in BPA-free containers.

Savory Broth

Turning your favorite food into a soup by adding water makes it more filling, and you eat fewer calories; adding broth makes it even better. Broth can also be enjoyed as a hot beverage alternative to lattes or other fattening coffee drinks.

INGREDIENTS

1 to 2 pounds (455 to 905 g) of meat with bones (chicken, beef, or other meat)

2 large carrots, cut into pieces

1 large onion, cut into pieces

2 large stalks of celery, cut into pieces (or 1 cup chopped celery ribs with leaves)

½ teaspoon salt

1 teaspoon pepper or 8 to 10 whole peppercorns

1 or 2 bay leaves

1 to 2 teaspoons chopped parsley, rosemary, thyme, or any other herb or spice combination you desire (optional)

DIRECTIONS

Add meat with bones (no skin), vegetables, salt, pepper, herbs, and bay leaf into a large stockpot and cover with 8 cups (1.9 L) of cold filtered water. Bring to a boil and immediately reduce heat. Simmer uncovered or partially covered for three to four hours (longer cooking time for stronger broth). Set aside until cool enough to handle. Strain and keep the broth. Discard all solid pieces. Cover the broth and store it in the refrigerator overnight. Next morning, remove any fat that has congealed at the top. Chicken and beef broth should have a gelatinous consistency when cold because of the high protein content. Reheat and enjoy.

NUTRITIONAL INFO

Broth has only 8 calories per cup, and that comes from a gram of protein and a gram of carbohydrates.

Fill Up First on Low-Calorie Foods

Start your dinner with a big salad, a large bowl of healthy soup, or a full serving of vegetables (or all three!). This fills up your stomach with low-calorie foods and gets your gut hormones working to shut down your appetite so you end up eating less of the higher calorie foods.

Dr. Barbara Rolls from Penn State studied preschool-age children and showed that serving vegetables as a first course can be a very effective way to increase vegetable consumption.

Most Popular Beans to Cook from Scratch

KIDNEY BEANS

The deep red color of kidney beans is a source of antioxidants and other beneficial phytochemicals. They are very sturdy, meaning they don't fall apart easily, and are a good bean to try for first-time bean chefs. Kidney beans are excellent eaten alone or can be used in hot or cold dishes such as chili, soups, stews, and bean salad.

BLACK BEANS

My personal favorite, black beans, have a distinctive yet mild flavor that goes great with metabolism-boosting hot sauce.

PINTO BEANS

Pinkish brown and mild in flavor, pinto beans are full of nutrients and fiber, and easy to find in just about any grocery store.

CHICKPEAS (GARBANZO BEANS)

A round bean with a nutty flavor, chickpeas are very filling. Serve hot as a dish or in soup or cold in a salad. Smash them into a creamy dense paste to make hummus.

ADUKI BEANS

A smaller red bean that is sweet and nutty tasting, they are an excellent substitute for meat and can be eaten as a meal with vegetables and a starch. They are popular in Asian cooking, and good when you are working on increasing the variety of healthy foods in your diet. Because of their smaller size, they only need to soak for an hour or less before cooking.

WHITE BEANS

Soak larger white beans for seven to eight hours before cooking. White beans can be puréed or smashed into a hummus-like paste and used as a dip or a substitute for mashed potatoes, or they can be used whole in soups and salads.

FINALLY LEARN HOW TO COOK BEANS

Beans are one of the healthiest foods you can eat. I recommend learning how to make dried beans from scratch. There is a short learning curve, but once mastered, you will be amazed at how easy it can be. An added benefit is that dried beans are much cheaper than canned beans.

Canned beans are fine if you don't have the time, but if you want to avoid the sodium, preservatives, and BPA exposures (even from organic canned beans) and explore tasty new varieties of beans, then dried beans are the best.

Don't Get Too Creative

When soaking beans, do not add salt or anything acidic (such as tomatoes or vinegar), as it makes the skin of the bean tough to chew.

Soak Beans Before You Cook Them

The key to successfully cooking dried beans is soaking them before cooking. The larger the bean, the longer you have to soak them.

The average bean needs to soak for about six hours, not overnight. Read the package for exact times. Regardless of the size of the bean, the longer you soak them, the shorter time it will take to cook them.

If beans give you an upset stomach, try soaking them for 30 to 45 minutes longer to allow the starches more time to break down. Soaking the beans makes them expand with water, increasing bulk, weight, and volume. This shuts off hunger and makes you feel full and satisfied.

Step by Step: Cooking Dried Beans from Scratch

- Try different varieties of organic dried beans—you might even ask your grocer to special-order varieties they don't normally stock. Be sure to check the freshness date (some natural food stores sell bulk beans that can get old).
- Pour the beans into a large, shallow container so you can easily spot and remove any stones or small shriveled beans. Transfer the beans to a colander and rinse, removing any remaining little stones.
- Place beans back in the container, add 3 to 4 cups (710 to 950 ml) of filtered water for every cup of beans, and cover with a lid. Soak small beans for 6 to 7 hours, medium beans for 6 to 8 hours, and large beans for 8 to 9 hours.
- Strain, rinse, and discard extra water before cooking. The hydrated beans should be three times their original size (i.e., 1 cup of dry beans should expand to 3 cups of hydrated beans).
- Use a cast-iron, stainless steel, or cast-aluminum pot. Add 10 cups (2.4 L) of fresh, filtered water to the cooking pot, and add the beans. Bring to a boil, lower the heat, cover, and simmer for 60 to 90 minutes until the beans are tender (specific times will be listed on the package). Do not bring the water back to boil; keep it simmering to prevent the beans from breaking when they cook.
- Add flavorings, herbs, and spices (1 to 2 teaspoons per 1 pound [0.5 kg] of beans), such as garlic, black pepper, cumin, or chili powder, about 30 to 45 minutes before the beans finish cooking. Explore bean dish recipes, such as Boston baked beans or Spanish black beans, in books, magazines, and on the Internet.
- Remove from heat, cool, store, or serve and enjoy!

Hearty Protein and Bean Soup

This basic recipe can be turned into many different soups. Try a variety of proteins, beans, and seasonings to create different varieties. This soup is great for lunch, dinner, or an afternoon snack. It's also a great food to fight cravings for salty carbohydrates, as I discuss in chapter 4. This recipe makes four servings.

INGREDIENTS

- 1 teaspoon olive oil
- 1 large onion, cut into small pieces
- 1 large carrot, chopped
- 1 to 2 tablespoons (5 to 10 g) chopped herbs
- 2 cups (475 ml) broth or stock (chicken, beef, vegetable)
- 1 cup (150 g) cooked protein, cut into small pieces (chicken breast, turkey breast, shrimp, lean beef, pork, lamb, etc.)
- 1½ cups (150 g) cooked beans (kidney, black, navy, garbanzo, etc.)

DIRECTIONS

Heat oil in a large pot over medium-high heat. Add onions and carrots. Cook, stirring often, until soft, 3 to 4 minutes. Add in chopped herbs and cook about 1 minute until you begin to smell the herbs. Add broth, cover, and increase the temperature to high, bringing to a boil. Add the cooked protein and beans. Stir occasionally for 3 to 4 minutes, then cool to store or serve hot.

NUTRITIONAL INFO

For each serving (approx. ¼ of recipe):
Calories: 150 | Carbohydrates: 26 g | Protein: 25 g | Fat: 4 g | Fiber: 5 g

Protein and Vegetable Soup

This basic recipe can also be turned into many different soups. Try a variety of proteins, vegetables, herbs, and seasonings. This soup is great for lunch, dinner, or an afternoon snack. It's also great for fighting salty carb cravings. Makes four servings.

INGREDIENTS

1 teaspoon olive oil

2 cups (160 g) cut-up vegetables

1 to 2 tablespoons (5 to 10 g) chopped herbs

2 cups (475 ml) broth or stock (chicken, beef, vegetable)

1 cup (150 g) cooked protein, cut into small pieces (chicken breast, turkey breast, lean beef, pork, lamb, etc.)

DIRECTIONS

Heat olive oil in a large pot over medium-high heat and add vegetables. Cook, stirring often, until soft, 3 to 4 minutes. Add chopped herbs and cook about 1 minute until you begin to smell the herbs. Add broth and protein, cover, and increase the temperature, bringing to a boil. Stir occasionally for 3 to 4 minutes, and then cool to store or serve hot.

NUTRITIONAL INFO

For each serving (approx. ¼ of recipe):
Calories: 240 | Carbohydrates: 20 g | Protein: 30 g | Fat : 4 g | Fiber: 5 g

Top Off a Good Day with Dessert

Treat yourself to a delicious, delectable sweet, slow-carbohydrate dessert every night. This helps satisfy your cravings for sweets and prevents blood sugar and insulin spikes. The slow carbohydrates help boost serotonin to help calm anxiety and help you have a deep, restful sleep.

Don't deprive yourself. Many people have said don't eat after a certain time, but I disagree with this advice. Eating a slow-carb dessert not only helps your hormones, but it gives you a sweet treat at the end of each day and should be something you enjoy and look forward to. This helps you stick with the BLADD all the way to the "enD" each day. See chapter 5 for more on desserts.

PRACTICE MAKES NEARLY PERFECT

As you practice the BON! Eating Plan, it will become an automatic part of your daily routine. Many of my patients tell me that they know this way of eating makes sense. They also know that eating perfectly is not possible over the long haul and that overeating often gets in the way following this plan day in and day out. That is where the rest of this book will help you to overcome the challenges of eating well-balanced meals on the BLADD schedule.

In part 2, I address the main problems that cause overeating, from cravings to a slow metabolism and chemical disruptors to your endocrine system. Once you understand how these problems influence your overeating, you can take charge of your life and return to a healthy, ideal weight.

The changes you make are intended to last forever, but that doesn't mean an eating life of drudgery. Instead, you will be nourished by a rainbow of fruits and vegetables, along with whole grains, lean meats, and lean dairy products.

In part 3, you'll learn about how your lifestyle can affect your hunger hormones, causing you to overeat. Good and bad behaviors such as exercise, sleeping, and mindless eating will be addressed to keep you on the BLADD schedule to beat overeating now!

BON! 7-day Meal Plan

In addition to the detailed recipes sprinkled throughout this chapter, you'll find great recipe ideas by searching these menu items on the Internet.

DAY 1

Breakfast	Lunch	Snack	Dinner	Dessert
2 or 3 chicken or turkey sausage links with 2 poached eggs	Chicken Italiano soup	Slices of turkey with mustard	Veggie shrimp stir-fry	Low-fat yogurt with fruit
1 medium grapefruit			Large salad	

DAY 2

Breakfast	Lunch	Snack	Dinner	Dessert
Omelet made with 4 egg whites, 1 egg yolk, and 2 ounces (55 g) of chopped chicken or ham	Large salad with protein	Boiled shrimp	Grilled chicken breast	High-fiber breakfast cereal with fruit and skim milk
1 cup (160 g) of cubed cantaloupe or honeydew	1 cup (145 g) of strawberries		Vegetables	
			Baked potato	

DAY 3

Breakfast	Lunch	Snack	Dinner	Dessert
16-ounce (475 ml) smoothie	Sandwich made with 3 to 4 ounces (85 to 115 g) lean protein, lettuce, and tomato on whole-grain bread	Celery sticks filled with fat-free cream cheese, topped with crushed nuts	Grilled fish	Low-calorie frozen dessert treat
1 string cheese	1 medium banana		Corn on the cob	
			Brown rice	
			Large salad	

DAY 4

Breakfast	Lunch	Snack	Dinner	Dessert
1 to 2 cups (230 to 460 g) of Greek yogurt topped with ½ cup (40 g) high-fiber breakfast cereal	Whole-wheat pasta with vegetables (sautéed or raw) and chopped chicken or beef	Smoothie	Beans and rice	Fruit and low-fat cheese
Hard-boiled egg	Watermelon		Steamed vegetables	
1 cup (145 g) of mixed berries			Large salad	

DAY 5

Breakfast	Lunch	Snack	Dinner	Dessert
1 cup (225 g) of fat-free cottage cheese topped with ½ cup (80 g) of chopped pineapple	Frozen, low-calorie entrée and package of frozen vegetables	Cut-up pieces of cooked chicken breast	Large bowl of soup with protein, vegetables, and potatoes	Smoothie
Hard-boiled egg			Green salad with crushed nuts and low-fat cheese	2 squares of dark chocolate
1 slice of whole-grain toast			Large salad	

DAY 6

Breakfast	Lunch	Snack	Dinner	Dessert
6 ounces (170 g) of steel-cut oatmeal	Baked potato topped with turkey chili	Hard-boiled egg	Shrimp and vegetable kabobs	Pineapple cubes
2 ounces (55 g) of sliced turkey or ham	Sliced peaches		Sweet potato	Fat-free cottage cheese
1 cup (150 g) of fruit salad				

DAY 7

Breakfast	Lunch	Snack	Dinner	Dessert
6 scrambled egg whites with 1 or 2 yolks, mixed with unlimited chopped vegetables	Grilled salmon (cold or hot) with vegetables	Beef jerky	Turkey meatloaf	Strawberries dipped in melted dark chocolate. (Stick with 3 or 4 chocolate-covered strawberries and if you are still hungry, eat more plain ones.)
Sliced orange	1 cup (145 g) blueberries		Quinoa	Fat-free cottage cheese
			Spinach salad	

Chicken Italiano Soup

This delicious and filling soup recipe makes four servings.

INGREDIENTS

2 teaspoons (10 ml) olive oil

1 clove garlic, chopped

2 cups (360 g) diced tomatoes

2 cups (430 g) white beans, cooked

2 cups (475 ml) chicken broth

1 cup (140 g) cooked chicken breast meat

1 cup (140 g) cooked whole-wheat elbow macaroni

1 cup (30 g) fresh baby spinach

1 tablespoon (2.5 g) chopped fresh basil

1 tablespoon (4 g) chopped fresh oregano

4 tablespoons (20 g) grated Parmesan cheese

DIRECTIONS

Add oil to pot with garlic and simmer for 1 minute. Then add the tomatoes, beans, and broth, and bring to a boil over high heat. Reduce heat, cover, and simmer for 6 minutes. Add the chicken, macaroni, spinach, basil, and oregano, and simmer for 2 to 3 minutes. To serve, top with 1 tablespoon (4 g) Parmesan cheese.

NUTRITIONAL INFO

Per serving (1 cup)
Calories: 200 | Carbohydrates: 21 g | Fiber: 4 g | Protein: 18 g | Fat: 5 g

Tasty Turkey Chili

This hearty chili recipe makes four servings.

INGREDIENTS

1 tablespoon (15 ml) olive oil

1 pound (455 g) ground turkey breast

2 cups (500 g) kidney beans, cooked

1 cup (180 g) diced tomatoes

1 clove garlic, chopped

1 cup (150 g) chopped green bell pepper

2 tsp (5 g) chili powder

1 tsp ground cumin

¼ cup (60 ml) water

DIRECTIONS

Heat a large pan over medium heat, then add the olive oil. Brown the ground turkey, stirring constantly for 3 to 4 minutes until done. Add the kidney beans, tomatoes, garlic, bell pepper, chili powder, cumin, and water and bring to a boil. Simmer for 10 minutes. Cool and enjoy.

NUTRITIONAL INFO

Per serving (1 cup)

Calories: 213 | Fat: 5 g | Carbohydrates: 23 g | Fiber: 7 g | Protein: 19 g

Make More Than You Need and Store

It's smart to make a large batch because you can store some for later. Most meals are fine in the refrigerator for three to four days and in a freezer for up to six months when frozen in BPA-free storage containers.

PART TWO:
Details Behind the Eating Plan That Will Keep You on Track

Turn Off Your Appetite

Your appetite is all in your mind, literally. It's your brain's way of controlling your weight. Think of the brain as the master control center, sensing what the body needs in terms of fuel and sending messages to the body to act. Hunger is a brain process, driven by what I call "hunger hormones" because they send signals to the brain to turn your appetite on or off. All overeating is linked to the brain.

Is Your Appetite Out of Control?

___ Do you get hungrier after you start eating?
___ Do you skip breakfast?
___ Do you feel hungry when you shouldn't?
___ Is food a primary source of pleasure in your life?
___ Have you had periods of time when you went more than twenty-four hours without eating any healthy food?
___ Do you have trouble sticking to a diet for more than a few days?
___ Do you lose weight slowly then regain weight quickly?
___ Do you plateau before reaching your goal weight when on a diet?
___ Does the scale stay in the same place no matter what you do?
___ Do you use fat substitutes or drink diet soda?

If you answered yes to any of these questions, you can get help by following the Action Plan in this chapter.

***action*plan**

Control Your Appetite

- *Avoid appetite stimulators.*
- *Start the day with a big high-protein breakfast.*
- *Eat meals and snacks on a schedule.*
- *Use variety and monotony to your advantage.*
- *Eat comfort foods at dinner with extra vegetables.*
- *Use vinegar to control your appetite.*
- *Don't use fat substitutes or drink diet soda.*
- *Take vitamin D.*
- *Plan rewards.*
- *Drink coffee or tea.*

Understand How Some Foods Make You Hungry

Some foods put your appetite in the wrong direction. While the right kind of food makes you feel full and satisfied, appetite-stimulating foods do the opposite. This is why you may feel hungrier after you start eating particular foods. Have you ever wondered why they call it an appetizer? Although I always encourage focusing on a "to-do" approach, this is a situation where you need to put a few items on your "not to-do" list.

Appetite-stimulating foods have either a short-term or long-term effect. Short-term appetite stimulators are the appetizers, salty snacks, alcohol, and other foods that make you hungrier for more food. Long-term appetite stimulators pose a more serious danger, and include unhealthy foods (especially high-fat foods) that are eaten consistently on a day-to-day basis.

UNHEALTHY FOODS MAKE YOU WANT TO EAT MORE

Eating unhealthy foods on a chronic basis can boost your appetite over time. You should never go more than twenty-four hours without eating healthy foods. Even if you are in a situation where healthy food is hard to come by, make every effort to get some healthy food every twenty-four hours. Eating primarily unhealthy food for more than twenty-four hours will turn on appetite centers in your brain that tend to stay on for a long time.

The Best and Worst Snacks for Weight Loss

It's time to give up potato chips. A 2011 Harvard study published in the *New England Journal of Medicine* found that chips are the worst snacks to eat if you're trying to lose weight. Other foods sure to put on the pounds include sweetened beverages (including diet soda) and red meat.

The study also found that yogurt was the best snack for losing weight, preventing about 0.8 pound (0.4 kg) of weight gain in a four-year period. Fruits, vegetables, and whole grains also scored well. The Harvard study also found that sleeping six to eight hours per night was ideal for weight loss (see chapter 10).

Avoid Appetite Stimulators

Appetite stimulators trigger cravings and hunger. These snacks are high in calories, sugar, and fat, and are low in volume. They tend to send your appetite soaring. You should replace or dilute appetite-stimulating foods with low-calorie foods.

APPETITE STIMULATOR	TRY THIS INSTEAD
Nuts	Use nuts as a topping or part of a recipe
Cheese	Eat tiny amounts with a piece of fruit, or in a vegetable dish
Dried fruit	Fresh fruit
Restaurant appetizer	Bowl of soup
Chips and salsa	Celery sticks filled with fat-free cream cheese
Pretzels	Carrot sticks and hummus
Bread and butter	Hard-boiled egg
Candy	Dark chocolate
Soda	Iced tea with lemon
Alcoholic drinks	Diet tonic water* or club soda with lemon

*Even though diet tonic water contains artificial sweeteners, the bitter flavor helps calm appetite instead of boosting it like diet sodas do.

Start the Day with a Big High-Protein Breakfast

In my first book, *Hormonal Balance*, published in 2002, I emphasized the importance of starting the day with a protein-rich breakfast. This advice is now a "must do," recommended by almost every nutrition expert I know. Eggs are a great protein breakfast, especially egg whites, but many of my patients have told me that they can't eat an egg white omelet every day. Other good choices include turkey sausages, yogurt, and cottage cheese (see chapter 2 for more ideas).

Protein is a critical component to a balanced breakfast. Protein suppresses ghrelin, a hunger hormone (see chapter 6) and prevents insulin spikes (see chapter 5). High-carbohydrate breakfasts, such as a bagel with fat-free cream cheese, toast and jelly, or cereal and skim milk, will cause your blood sugar and insulin to surge, making you ravenous late in the morning or just before lunch. Insulin is a hunger hormone that spikes any time sugar levels rise in your blood.

BENEFITS BACKED BY RESEARCH

A big breakfast with protein will help reduce your appetite at both lunch and dinner, lowering your overall calories for the day. Think of it as investing calories in the morning to save calories later.

In the Big Breakfast Study conducted by Dr. Daniela Jakubowicz in 2007, participants who ate a big breakfast with a lot of protein were able to lose weight and keep it off without feeling hungry or having cravings. Another study from The Netherlands compared the hormonal effects of a high-protein breakfast (with about 60 percent protein) with a lower protein breakfast (20 percent protein). The high-protein breakfast caused a more robust decrease in ghrelin levels and boosted a number of antihunger hormones, including cholecystokinin and glucagon-like peptide 1.

Eat Meals and Snacks on a Schedule

Plan the times when you will eat all your meals and snacks. Write it down and do everything you can to stick to your plan. Make sure you plan for a big breakfast, a healthy balanced lunch, a protein-rich afternoon snack, a veggie-packed dinner, and a slow-carb dessert. If you need to, set an alarm on your phone. Being healthy takes work, but planning your meals and snacks will make your life much easier in the long run.

Researchers at Tufts University found that planning meals in advance is one of the most effective strategies for weight loss. Eating on a schedule helps you prevent swings in hunger hormones, which I discuss at length in chapter 6, and keeps your appetite lower throughout the day.

DON'T ALLOW YOURSELF TO GET HUNGRY

I am telling you that you must not let yourself get hungry. When you are hungry, you don't have willpower. It is much harder to eat healthy foods when you are very hungry because high ghrelin and low leptin levels make you crave high-calorie foods. When you are hungry, your hormones are out of control, and you are much more likely to overeat unhealthy foods.

By eating on a schedule, you can avoid extreme hunger that makes you more likely to eat an unhealthy snack or pig out at the next meal. Eating on a schedule takes planning to make it happen well. If you don't plan, you'll find yourself in situations where you don't have the tools you need (healthy foods) to get your job done.

RECOGNIZE HOW THE BRAIN TAKES ALL

The brain is selfish. Sensing that you haven't eaten for a while, it does what it can to preserve itself by feeding off the remaining nutrients in your body. This results in a decrease in functioning of the other organs. Ultimately, your metabolism slows. The result is that you feel tired, or have brain fog. When you give the brain a continuous source of food, it functions at peak performance, boosting energy levels and cognitive functioning.

Use Variety and Monotony to Your Advantage

It's important to increase the variety of healthy foods you eat. Explore different types of fruits and vegetables and new healthy dishes. Try different healthy foods for breakfast and lunch. Especially make an effort to increase variety at breakfast, a time when most people tend to be fairly monotonous.

You can beat overeating at dinner by having a fairly monotonous meal then. This doesn't mean you have to eat the same meal every night. Choose three or four favorite healthy main dishes (see chapter 2) and rotate them, combining different vegetables. Enjoy variety at dinner with new vegetables and salads.

Variety increases your appetite for those new foods. By increasing the variety of healthy foods you eat, you feel hungrier for these foods, helping you feel full on fewer calories.

Monotony decreases appetite. Studies in rats showed that rats fed a "normal" human diet gained a lot of weight compared to rats that were fed rat chow. Eating the same food can seem boring, but it does decrease your appetite.

Eat Comfort Foods at Dinner, with Extra Vegetables

Comfort foods don't have to be unhealthy foods. Try macaroni and cheese with blended cauliflower and broccoli, veggie lasagna, turkey meatloaf or any healthy version of your favorite comfort foods. My friend B. Smith likes to do "makeover" with a favorite meal, making a traditionally unhealthy meal into a healthy version. Imagine eating a gourmet healthy lasagna and tiramisu prepared by a master chef. Try new recipes and new versions of your favorite foods.

Definitely add several servings of vegetables to your dinner. You should have at least two or three servings; add a salad if necessary.

WHY YOU OVEREAT AT DINNER

Your appetite tends to be highest at dinnertime. The body craves foods that are heavy and satisfying at this time of the day. If you eat a dinner that is too light, you will have rebound hunger a few hours later. Comfort foods tend to make us feel full and satisfied. They also help us feel relaxed, lowering cortisol levels.

Don't Overdo It with Vinegar

Although I don't recommend drinking vinegar, you may mix a spoonful of vinegar in a glass of water and drink it when you need to turn off your appetite. Vinegar is very acidic, so never drink it undiluted. Drinking excessive amounts can cause bone loss and other health problems, so you should keep it to less than 3 to 4 tablespoons (45 to 60 ml) of vinegar per day.

Use Vinegar to Control Your Appetite

For centuries, vinegar has been touted as a remedy to cure almost any ailment. Even today, vinegar is used as a weight-loss agent and body cleanser by alternative medicine practitioners.

Indeed, research has proven that vinegar suppresses appetite. In one study, participants who consumed vinegar along with white bread felt more full and satisfied than when they ate the white bread alone. That's because vinegar slows digestion and enhances satiety, a concept I discuss in chapter 6. Other research has shown that vinegar reduces blood sugar and insulin spikes, especially with high-carbohydrate foods.

The active ingredient in vinegar is acetic acid. Stronger tasting vinegars that contain a lot of acetic acid are the best at suppressing appetite.

USE VINEGAR EVERY DAY

Try using vinegar in your cooking and on salads every day. This is a good area to increase variety and sample new things; explore different types, such as balsamic, apple cider, red wine, or rice vinegar. I recommend using a vinegar and oil set but filling both bottles with different types of vinegar, making it a vinegar and vinegar set.

Try Spicy, Pickled Vegetables

Spicy, pickled vegetables are a delicacy in many ethnic dishes. Just think about the benefits! Beyond tasting delicious, they fill you up and have a lot of vinegar to suppress your appetite. The spiciness helps speed up your metabolism too. A study from Ajou University School of Medicine in Korea found that eating the spicy fermented cabbage kimchi reduces body weight and improves metabolism.

Avoid Fat Substitutes and Artificial Sweeteners

Although you should eat foods that are low in fat and calories, that doesn't mean that foods containing synthetic substitutes are okay. Fat substitutes, such as olestra, and artificial sweeteners, such as those in diet soda, can backfire, causing increased appetite and carbohydrate cravings. When cooking, however, artificial sweeteners are okay in limited amounts.

SUBSTITUTES CONFUSE THE BRAIN

Even though foods made with synthetic fat substitutes have fewer calories than their full-fat versions, they can make you gain weight. Foods that merely *taste* fatty send a message to the brain that indicates a high number of calories. This triggers the body to react metabolically, increasing salivation and secreting hormones that trick the body. When the brain is misled by food that contains fewer calories than it appears to have, hunger increases, driving the body to seek out the missing calories.

Fat substitutes disrupt the relationship between the taste of food and the caloric impact. This causes a dysregulation of energy balance, leading to increased appetite and weight gain. Researchers at Purdue University examined the effects of the fat substitute olestra in rats by comparing the effects of regular potato chips and nonfat potato chips. Rats that ate the nonfat chips gained more weight than the rats that ate regular potato chips because the fat substitutes actually increased hunger, making the rats consume even more calories. The same researchers have reported similar findings in rats when they were given artificial sweeteners that promoted weight gain and increased body fat.

Plan Rewards for Your Healthy Behaviors

Many experts will tell you to use nonfood rewards, such as a new clothing item, a massage, or a car wash. Nonfood rewards are great, but it is okay for you to go ahead and use a special food or meal as a reward from time to time.

You deserve it! What's more, if you don't have small treats, you'll set yourself up for feelings of deprivation, binge eating, and possibly depression.

We all need rewards. Without any rewards, life is miserable. Many of my patients who follow a diet without rewards tell me that they feel depressed. Depressed people typically have an inability to experience pleasure, known as anhedonia. They feel as if they have suffered a loss, like a death of a loved one. But the loss is from missing favorite foods that give pleasure.

Eating healthy foods requires constant motivation and self-discipline . . . in other words, willpower. Eating unhealthy foods is easy, not stressful, and gives us a lot of pleasure. Unhealthy foods are easy to find, inexpensive, prepared, and taste delicious.

A continuous state of self-denial leads to feelings of deprivation, and a situation that is impossible to maintain. The dopamine reward system in the brain is so strong that it can overpower other hunger hormones and make you eat when you aren't hungry.

UNDERSTAND THAT STRESS DESTROYS WILLPOWER

When you force your body into a rigid lifestyle, it can leave you feeling burned out and vulnerable to temptation. Add more life stress, and your willpower can crack. It doesn't matter what type of stress we endure, the stress from dieting or the stress from life, our bodies can only take so much. Too much stress from one area makes it difficult to endure stress in another.

Many of my patients have told me they just can't stand the thought of not eating their favorite food or going to a special restaurant with friends. One of my patients told me that losing his favorite candy bar was like losing a friend. Adding an occasional reward works to reduce the stress of strict eating, allowing you to continue your healthy lifestyle for the long haul.

HOW MUCH SHOULD YOU SPLURGE?

The reward needs to be something you look forward to for a long time and have to work hard for. Your reward should not be a whole day or a whole weekend of binge eating. The reward should also be reasonable enough so that it doesn't counteract an entire week of healthy eating.

You must plan your reward well in advance and write it down. While you're at it, write down what you are going to do to earn the reward. For example, if you eat healthy foods and exercise every day this week, you will eat dinner at your favorite restaurant on Saturday night. The reward should be a specific meal or a specific food.

Double or Triple the Dose, Depending on Weight

Endocrinologists have identified the close link of vitamin D to obesity and agree that having normal vitamin D levels is a necessary step for losing weight and maintaining a healthy weight. However, in June 2011, Dr. Michael Holick, an endocrinologist and the guru of vitamin D, presented new guidelines at the prestigious Endocrine Society meeting in Boston, Massachusetts. People who are overweight or obese require double or triple the standard dose of vitamin D, Dr. Holick concluded.

Take Plenty of Vitamin D

Our skin makes natural vitamin D when exposed to the sun. However, most people today do not get much exposure to sunlight, due to our modern lifestyle and use of sunscreens. Over the last few years, vitamin D deficiency has emerged as a serious medical problem, closely linked to body weight and body fat. Although it is called a vitamin, vitamin D acts like a hormone in every sense, transmitting the body's signals through the bloodstream to target receptors scattered throughout the body.

I don't suggest sunbathing because of the increased risk for skin cancer. Instead, I recommend that you take 2000 to 4000 IU of vitamin D every day. For children, the dose should be 400 to 600 IU. The heavier you are, the more vitamin D you need to take. The foods you eat usually don't supply enough vitamin D. A serving of fish contains 300 to 400 IU; a cup of milk has 100 IU. Vitamin D_3, or cholecalciferol, is available without a prescription and comes from a natural source, cod liver oil.

Studies have shown that the more you weigh, the lower your vitamin D level. Presumably, the reason for this is that excess body fat sequesters vitamin D, a fat-soluble vitamin. The more fat in your body, the more vitamin D gets hidden in fat, where your body can't use it. Vitamin D plays a role in a wide spectrum of diseases, from high blood pressure to diabetes and cancer. We are only just starting to learn the importance of vitamin D.

VITAL STATS FOR VITAMIN D

I check a vitamin D level as part of a standard evaluation in overweight and obese patients and have seen that 80 to 90 percent have levels lower than they should be. Large population studies back up this observation and have shown that most people are vitamin D deficient, even if they live in sunny areas. If vitamin levels are very low, I will prescribe a prescription form, Vitamin D_2, or ergocalciferol, which is available in very potent dosages for the first few months. The standard, over-the-counter doses of vitamin D can take many months or even years to fully replace depleted vitamin D reserves.

If you are more than 25 pounds (11 kg) overweight or have symptoms of vitamin D deficiency, such as bone pain, fatigue, or muscle weakness, you should see your physician to be tested for vitamin D deficiency.

Drink Coffee or Tea

Coffee and tea are healthy for you to drink. I wouldn't want you to overdose on caffeine, but there is no reason to limit coffee or tea from your life. Too much caffeine can cause insomnia, anxiety, nausea, high blood pressure, and other symptoms. You can enjoy either caffeinated or decaffeinated versions but should limit caffeinated servings to four cups daily.

It's smart to replace higher calorie beverages with coffee and tea. Beware of specialty coffees, which can be very high in calories, sugar, and fat. Try different types of tea, such as black tea, Earl Grey, or green tea. Try different types of coffee from around the world. Explore new recipes for low-calorie coffee and tea drinks.

COFFEE AND TEA ARE LOADED WITH ANTIOXIDANTS

Although many studies have shown that caffeine suppresses appetite and boosts metabolism, the real benefits from coffee and tea aren't from the caffeine. In fact, the health benefits of coffee and tea are seen with both caffeinated and decaffeinated versions.

Coffee and tea have huge amounts of antioxidants and other potent compounds. Coffee and tea have been shown to decrease the risk for diabetes, cancer, and many other ailments. These drinks have zero calories, and there are a lot of different types you can explore to add variety to your noncaloric beverages.

Drink Green Tea

Green tea has been shown in multiple studies to help with weight loss by speeding metabolism and helping the body burn fat. The metabolism boosting effect of green tea comes from compounds called catechin polyphenols, along with the caffeine.

Remember, the Brain Is in Charge

The brain listens to hormonal signals from the body, gathering information from the fat cells, the stomach and intestines, the liver, the pancreas, the thyroid, and the adrenal glands. It processes that information in the appetite

Choose Organic Coffee

Whenever possible, drink coffee from organically grown beans—that is, without pesticides. Coffee beans have a very thin skin and tend to take up a lot of chemicals that you can't wash off.

control center, known as the hypothalamus and arcuate nucleus, which then directs our behavior to eat, not to eat, or to overeat.

But the motivation for a healthy lifestyle comes from more than just the hypothalamus. Higher brain centers control "executive functions" that coordinate our behaviors. It is important to understand that the brain can cause you to overeat for many different reasons.

So many factors come into play as our brain regulates our eating behaviors. For example, if you force your body into a rigid lifestyle or put yourself on an ultrastrict diet, without taking time to reward yourself, even though you practice healthy behaviors, there is a chance your brain could revolt and you won't be able to stick to a diet for long or you will binge eat as your brain seeks the reward and pleasure it has been lacking. If the brain senses it is missing something, it will direct behaviors to seek food from the immediate environment, resulting in overeating and obesity.

Because the brain controls our eyesight, hearing, and senses of smell, taste, and touch, just the sight, smell, or even verbal descriptions of food can set off a cascade of hunger hormones that enable the body to prepare for food that it anticipates is on its way.

A Pleasure Center Gone Awry

The brain controls motivation, pleasure, and rewards. These higher brain functions have a lot to do with eating and can be the source of overeating. After all, food is pleasure and can be addictive, just like a drug. In fact, the brain pathways that transfer the addictive properties of drugs and alcohol are the same ones active in food addiction and compulsive overeating.

HOW HUNGER HORMONES OPERATE

All your hunger hormones affect your brain. Leptin, ghrelin, PYY, cortisol, thyroid hormone, estrogen, and testosterone all exert various effects by stimulating their respective receptors in the brain. Hormones affect the brain and the brain affects hormones; it goes both ways. When we understand what a hormone is and how it works, we access the key that unlocks the mystery of why we overeat.

Hunger hormones such as leptin are known to affect how our brain is motivated (or not motivated) to seek out healthy foods, or to exercise. It is known that leptin resistance, for example, results in decreased motivation to have healthy behaviors.

The brain hormones responsible for appetite are neuropeptide Y (NPY), serotonin, dopamine, and endocannabinoids. Brain hormones are also known as neurotransmitters. They are different than regular hormones because for the most part, they stay localized within the brain, sending messages to receptors there.

However, the brain hormones do circulate in the blood and thus have effects throughout the body, not just the brain. They can turn metabolism up or down and direct the body to store fat. For example, neuropeptide Y actually tells fat cells to grow and multiply.

Just Say No to Energy Drinks

You should avoid all energy drinks, even the diet versions. Diet energy drinks contain artificial sweeteners and a lot of caffeine. In addition to giving your body a temporary jolt from the caffeine, the sweet flavor sends a confusing message to your brain. Your brain prepares your body for sugar, and when the drink fails to satisfy, you start craving sugar for hours or days.

Neuropeptide Y: King of the Hunger Hormones

Neuropeptide Y is secreted by the hypothalamus, and is the most potent appetite stimulator in the body. It is known as an orexigenic hormone.

Medical Term: Orexigenic

(From the Greek *orexis*, meaning "appetite.") Any substance that stimulates appetite. (The opposite of anorectic, also known as *anorexigenic*. *An*- means "without.")

STEP BY STEP

Ways to Lower Levels of Neuropeptide Y

- Combat leptin resistance by eating a healthy balanced diet, getting daily exercise, and six to eight hours of quality sleep every night.
- Eat enough protein (see chapter 6). Low-protein diets have been shown to increase neuropeptide Y production.
- Eat 40 percent of your daily calories as carbohydrates, but no more. A study from Rockefeller University showed that high-carbohydrate diets boost neuropeptide Y production.
- Don't eat a high-fat diet (see chapter 7). A study from Charles University in Prague showed that high-fat diets raise neuropeptide Y levels.
- Don't deprive yourself. Food restriction is a potent stimulator of neuropeptide Y production.

Neuropeptide Y decreases the desire to exercise, making you want to remain sedentary. The hormone also has a direct effect on fat cells, where receptors are located, causing them to grow—especially abdominal fat. Neuropeptide Y has a circadian rhythm, with a daily pattern of rising during the day and falling at night. This is one of the reasons that not getting enough sleep boosts appetite.

Neuropeptide Y also encourages the infiltration of macrophages into fat. As I discuss in chapter 7, fat macrophages, known as adipose tissue macrophages, or ATMs, are a major source of inflammation in the body and the major cause of leptin and insulin resistance. In fact, neuropeptide Y has direct links to type 2 diabetes, insulin resistance, and the metabolic syndrome that is discussed in chapter 5.

EATING DISORDERS AND OTHER DISEASES LINKED TO NPY

It is thought that eating disorders, such as compulsive overeating, may be related to the body producing too much neuropeptide Y or being hypersensitive to its already powerful effects. Researchers also believe that people with anorexia nervosa may have acquired resistance to the effects of neuropeptide Y, dampening its hunger-stimulating effect.

The National Center for Biotechnology Information, U.S. National Library of Medicine reports that mutations in the neuropeptide Y gene are associated with high cholesterol, increased alcohol consumption, metabolic syndrome, and cardiovascular disease.

If the Brain Is CEO, the Hypothalamus Is Managing Director

At the seat of the brain's appetite center, the hypothalamus is ultimately responsible for our hunger drive. It also controls the pituitary gland, which is known as the "master gland" because it controls glands that produce metabolic hormones such as the thyroid gland, the adrenal glands, the ovaries, and testes.

WHY HUNGER MAKES US EAT

Scientists believe that neuropeptide Y may be what makes hunger feel uncomfortable to us. In fact, the discomfort of hunger is one of the most basic drives in all living beings. Neuropeptide Y is responsible for that primal hunger drive that exists in all living creatures.

Research in rats and other animals has shown that injections of neuropeptide Y stimulate appetite and increase food consumption. Studies in monkeys and mice show that repeated stress boosts neuropeptide Y levels. Eating a high-fat and high-sugar diet has also been shown to increase neuropeptide Y levels, as well as belly fat.

Artificial Sweeteners and Neuropeptide Y

One of the reasons postulated that artificial sweeteners cause weight gain is because they boost neuropeptide Y levels.

The Vicious Cycle of the "Fat Brain"

Neuropeptide makes fat grow, and fat makes leptin, which travels through the bloodstream and links with leptin receptors in the brain. Leptin shuts down neuropeptide Y production. If you have leptin resistance (see chapter 7), this cycle is disrupted and leptin can't properly shut down neuropeptide Y.

Serotonin Makes You Feel Blissfully Satisfied

Derived from the amino acid tryptophan (found in turkey and other foods that contain protein), serotonin makes us feel happy and content, thus its nickname as the happiness hormone. Serotonin is also linked to appetite control and is involved in hunger and carbohydrate cravings. It generates the calm feeling you get when you eat a sugary food in response to a carbohydrate craving.

Serotonin is affected by many popular antidepressants and antianxiety medications, which can cause either weight gain or weight loss. Researchers believe that bulimia and compulsive eating may be related to a dysregulation of serotonin production.

Serotonin is not just a brain hormone, but has important effects throughout the body. In addition to appetite regulation and carbohydrate cravings, serotonin is related to sleep, mood, memory, and muscle function. Eighty percent of the body's serotonin is produced by the gut and is vital for proper gut functioning. It is even important for the proper functioning of platelets, which are one of our body's natural blood clotting factors.

In Search of the Magic Bullet

A special receptor for serotonin known as the 5-HT_{2C} receptor is most closely tied to appetite control, and is a target for pharmaceutical companies developing weight-loss medications.

STEP BY STEP

Healthy Ways to Increase Serotonin

- Use bright lights in the morning and spend more time outdoors. Light therapy is used as a treatment for seasonal depression because it boosts brain serotonin levels.
- Keep a regular sleep and wake cycle. Disturbances in your circadian rhythm can lower serotonin levels.
- Think positively. One study showed that self-induced improvements in mood raise serotonin levels substantially.
- Do a good deed. Performing an act of kindness can help you feel happier and increases serotonin in the brain.
- Get in control of your life. People who are out of control feel helpless and depressed. Feeling in control not only boosts serotonin levels but helps you in countless other ways.
- Exercise. Among all the other benefits of exercise, which I discuss in chapter 9, exercise helps stimulate serotonin production.
- Eat healthy carbohydrates. Processed carbohydrates and sugar causes a temporary boost in serotonin followed by a crash.
- Eat turkey and dairy products. Turkey and dairy products are high in tryptophan, the building block for serotonin.

Dopamine Focuses on Pleasure

We are driven by the pleasure the food produces, not the nutritional value. Many people overeat because they crave this pleasure. Dopamine, another brain hormone involved in appetite regulation, is also involved in the reward system within the brain.

When you smell, see, or think about food, dopamine is released, increasing appetite for foods that taste good and give us pleasure. This is known as a hedonic signal because when food is rewarding, it typically means that we want and don't need a particular food. The pleasure we receive through food's effect on dopamine pales in comparison to anything else, including drugs and alcohol.

> ### The Smart Gut
>
> Your stomach and intestines have as many neurons and neurological connections as your brain. Many of the neurotransmitters of the brain also exist in the gut.

Research has shown that obese people have fewer receptors for dopamine that help with feelings of pleasure and satisfaction when they eat. Scientists believe that obese people eat more because they are trying to boost dopamine in the reward and pleasure pathways of their brains, similar to the way addicts need to take drugs.

People who become addicted to cocaine, alcohol, and other drugs do so because they either don't produce enough dopamine or their bodies aren't sensitive to its effects. It is thought that dopamine's role in obesity may also be linked to this system. In fact, addiction to food and addiction to drugs both have links to a dysfunctional dopamine reward system.

Dopamine is also responsible for brain control of body movement. Parkinson's disease is caused by problems with dopamine production.

BREAKING THE ADDICTION TO FOOD

The dopamine reward system is so powerful that it can circumvent many normal biologic cues to stop eating. Think about a situation where you had an uncontrollable craving for an unhealthy food. You may not even have felt hungry and you knew the food was unhealthy, but when you ate it, you enjoyed it and it made you feel good. That's dopamine working behind the scenes.

The Action Plan in this chapter, along with the advice throughout this book, will help you calm your dopamine system. Your brain will learn to stop relying on food as a primary source of pleasure.

STEP BY STEP

Healthy Ways to Regulate Dopamine

- Increase your consumption of apples, bananas, and watermelon. These three fruits are thought to help regulate dopamine levels.
- Don't eat a lot of sugar. Overconsumption of sweet foods can disrupt your dopamine reward system.
- Don't keep junk food around the house. Studies have shown that visual cues from unhealthy foods induce food-seeking behaviors via the dopamine pathway.
- Enjoy. Taking time for pleasure satisfies the dopamine reward system. Lack of enjoyment in life can cause you to seek out food as a substitute form of pleasure.

Endocannabinoids Give You the Munchies

Endocannabinoids are natural marijuana-like substances produced by the brain that are potent appetite stimulators. They are also involved in pain, mood, and memory. These substances work directly on the hypothalamus to stimulate appetite.

Drugs to block the effect of endocannabinoids were once intensively researched and thought to be the next cure for obesity. In clinical studies, the problem with these medications was that they caused many people to feel depressed, and some even committed suicide. The rate of depression was so high that most of the research in this area has been abandoned.

It turns out that leptin resistance causes the brain to produce excess amounts of endocannabinoids. So while medications to block endocannabinoids have too many side effects, alleviating leptin resistance, which I discuss in chapter 7, is a great way to lower endocannabinoid production without making you feel depressed.

Case Study: Forty-Eight Hours of Unhealthy Eating

This is a story of my patient, Maria, age forty-one and the mother of two children. She had a normal body weight, according to the charts, but wanted to lose the 14 pounds (6.4 kg) she had slowly gained since high school.

Maria had a fairly healthy diet and exercised a few times a week. Everything was going along pretty well and she was not having any major problems. Then she went on vacation and started eating unhealthy foods. Within forty-eight hours, she started craving high-calorie foods and ate three meals a day in restaurants for several days.

When she returned home, Maria felt horrible, as if she had a hangover: fatigue and brain fog. In a few short days, she had done long-term damage to her appetite control centers. Maria gained a few pounds in a short period of time and never took off the weight. She just got used to weighing a few pounds more. Her exercise slowed down, and she ate more unhealthy foods more often because she craved them. She slowly started gaining more weight. Maria became officially "overweight" and couldn't understand why she couldn't lose the weight. She didn't seem to be doing much differently, but the weight kept packing on.

I performed a full medical evaluation and found everything to be normal. By this time, Maria needed to lose 25 pounds (11 kg), a seemingly impossible task.

Long story short, she followed the plan in this book and lost the 25 pounds (11 kg) in about six months and has been keeping it off. She is really happy now and looks back at how her eating and exercise habits slowly went down the tubes. The changes were so subtle over such a long period of time that she'd been oblivious.

What's New: Eat to Fuel "Good" Macrophages and Beat Disease

Macrophages are the latest subject in obesity research. They are considered a type of white blood cell, but they exist in many places other than the blood, including the brain.

Some macrophages begin their lives in the walls of the intestines, in an area called Peyer's patches, and take up small amounts of the foods we eat by a process known as phagocytosis, similar to the way an amoeba takes food. They eventually leave the intestines and travel through the bloodstream to invade and intermingle with the tissues and organs of our body. Macrophages live within the cells of organs, and are ultimately responsible for many of their functions and dysfunctions.

Hormones are chemical messengers, while macrophages are cellular messengers. Hormones ebb and flow, have diurnal rhythms, and can be higher or lower, moment to moment. You can take a hormone pill or shot and have a higher hormone level in an instant. You can't say that about macrophages. These cellular messengers are in it for the long haul. They don't change quickly.

WHEN THEY'RE BAD, THEY'RE REALLY BAD

It is clear that these complex cells play a critical role as the body's number one source of inflammation-causing chemicals, called cytokines. As I discuss in chapter 7, inflammation is caused by macrophages that invade fat tissue (known as adipose tissue macrophages, or ATMs). This is the main cause of leptin resistance and a reason body weight can get stuck at a higher set point.

These bad boys are why 98 percent of people who lose weight ultimately gain it back. Brain macrophages flip on the appetite switch, even when it should be off. Chronic, low-grade brain inflammation, caused by brain macrophages, results in dysfunctional appetite control.

POTENTIAL CANCER KILLERS THAT WORK AS WELL AS YOU EAT

Macrophages are considered immune system cells because they fight infections and cancer by engulfing harmful particles and digesting them. But these multifunctional cells have many more roles. They travel throughout the body and secrete inflammatory chemicals in almost every organ in the body, including the brain and fat cells. So macrophages can be good or bad.

The latest research has shown that macrophages are influenced by the contents they come in contact with. What does that mean? Let's just focus on macrophages that live in the wall of the intestines. They absorb the food you eat every day, engulfing tiny particles going through your digestive tract.

Science now shows that good food makes these cells turn into "good macrophages" and bad food does what you would expect. Bad macrophages are a serious problem when it comes to long-term weight management. The problem comes when bad macrophages leave the intestinal lining, go into the bloodstream, and travel to your brain and fat cells to set up shop.

For permanent weight loss, it is mandatory for you to understand and replace your bad macrophages with good macrophages. You need to replace the toxic cells with good macrophages that will help you keep your body weight at a healthy, normal level. Otherwise, your weight loss is likely to be temporary. Let me explain more.

ABLE TO GO FROM GOOD TO BAD IN THE COURSE OF A DAY

Research in animals has shown that when fed a high-fat diet, macrophages become predominantly "bad" within twenty-four hours. These macrophages move from the intestinal wall to the bloodstream and then, among other places, to the fat and to the brain.

In the brain, macrophages are known as microglia. Microglia hang out in the main hunger center of the brain, the arcuate nucleus. Bad macrophages that become "bad microglia" switch on the hunger center and keep it on. These invaders damage the appetite control center to make a person feel hungry all the time and crave high-calorie, high-fat foods.

In other words, eating a lot of unhealthy food causes brain damage. This is what is going on with most of us. Once the macrophages become bad microglia, they are in your brain for a long time. They create inflammation by pumping out inflammatory chemicals. Inflammation is ultimately what is responsible for keeping the appetite switch turned on even when it should shut off.

Even if you lose a little weight, the microglia keep the pressure on, making you feel hungrier. They are pumping out inflammation chemicals that do permanent damage to your arcuate nucleus. There is no science yet to back up my theory, but I suspect that the 2 percent of people who lose weight and keep it off permanently are the ones who learned to replace their bad microglia with good microglia.

The key is to remember how the invader macrophage works as a messenger. Macrophages are extremely sensitive to whether or not you are eating healthy foods. Even twenty-four hours of unhealthy eating is enough to start turning them bad. You must begin to eat more healthy foods and never go for an entire twenty-four-hour period eating unhealthy foods.

Even if you are in a situation where healthy food is scarce, you need to make sure you get some veggies and fruits, just to prevent this twenty-four-hour thing from happening. My advice throughout this book is prioritized to help you transform your macrophages and beat overeating for life.

CHAPTER 4

Curb Cravings

Cravings can derail even the best intentions to beat overeating. Many of my patients tell me stories about how out of control they feel when they have a craving. They know they shouldn't be eating that food, but they do it anyway; then they feel guilty.

A craving is an intense desire to eat a particular food. The difference between hunger and a craving is that a craving is for a specific food or type of food and hunger is increased appetite in general.

From a biological perspective, the two main causes of cravings are hormone disruptions and missing micronutrients. Hormone disruptions that lead to food cravings commonly arise from eating certain foods that set up a viscous cycle, making us crave that food. Premenstrual Syndrome food cravings, on the other hand, come from normal hormonal cycles of estrogen and progesterone that can be treated by predicting and eating for the craving.

*action*plan

Kiss Cravings Goodbye

- *Eat a variety of colors of vegetables and fruits.*
- *Avoid sugars and processed carbohydrates.*
- *Don't eat fake food.*
- *Add a morning snack for afternoon and evening cravings.*
- *Beat salty carbohydrate cravings with soup.*
- *Prevent carbohydrate cravings with protein.*
- *Prepare for premenstrual cravings.*
- *Exercise in the morning or at lunchtime to beat late-day cravings.*
- *Improve the duration and quality of your sleep.*
- *Create a diversion.*

Are Your Cravings Biological or Psychological?

Some cravings are not caused by biology, but by psychology. The more specific the food craving, especially cravings for unhealthy foods, the less likely it is caused by a biological problem. For example, a craving for barbecue potato chips or fudge swirl ice cream is probably not caused by a hormone problem or missing micronutrient, but more likely psychological pseudohunger triggered by emotions or a situation. This is an issue I discuss in chapter 11.

Cravings that come from missing micronutrients are easily solved. These cravings seem to come from nowhere and can be for just about anything. A micronutrient is a vitamin, mineral, phytochemical, antioxidant, or any other beneficial substance that is contained in fruits and vegetables and other natural foods. It is hard to list all the beneficial micronutrients contained in natural foods, but suffice it to say there are thousands. If you are missing any one of these, the result can be a craving.

It's important to recognize the difference between biological cravings and psychological cravings. This chapter addresses biological cravings caused by disrupted hormones and missing micronutrients.

Do You Crave:

___ Sugar or sweets?
___ Salty carbohydrates, chips, pretzels, or snack foods?
___ Unusual foods?
___ Unhealthy foods?
___ Chocolate?
___ Do you have cravings in the afternoon or evening?
___ Are your cravings associated with PMS?
___ Do you overeat foods you crave and then don't eat enough healthy foods?
___ Do you eat fewer than thirty-five servings of vegetables and fruits each week?
___ Do you suffer from lack of sleep?

If you answered yes to any of these questions, you can get help from the Action Items in this chapter.

Eat a Variety of Colors of Vegetables and Fruits

No vitamin pill can replicate all the nutrients contained in fruits and vegetables. Fruits and vegetables are packed full of antioxidants, substances that are critical for reducing inflammation, the primary cause of leptin resistance (chapter 6) and insulin resistance (chapter 5). Eating a lot of antioxidants is a critical step to beating overeating.

Bottom line, you must eat at a minimum of thirty-five servings of vegetables and fruits every week, which is five servings per day. A serving is about 1 cup of raw food or ½ cup of cooked. I consider this number an absolute minimum. You need to eat a variety of vegetables and fruits representing all the colors of the rainbow. Don't stick to just a few vegetables and fruits. Broaden your scope and increase variety by sampling as many as you can find.

It is better to double this number and eat five servings of vegetables and five servings of fruit on a daily basis. This may seem like a lot of vegetables and fruit, but I assure you this is not an excessive amount. Eating more vegetables and fruits is a surefire way to decrease appetite and cravings and help you beat overeating.

The Rainbow's Invisible Nutrient

I remember learning about the colors of the rainbow in my sixth-grade science class. ROY-G-BIV: red, orange, yellow, green, blue, indigo, and violet. After violet comes ultraviolet (UV), an invisible light that transmits energy in the form of radiation. UV light provides a missing nutrient that you don't get from eating your colors, vitamin D.

Even when you eat enough vegetables and fruits every day, you won't consume adequate amounts of vitamin D. Nature intended us to get vitamin D from that invisible part of the rainbow, but here is a time when I recommend against doing it nature's way. I don't advise you to get vitamin D from exposing yourself to the sun because I don't want you to increase your risk for skin cancer. The answer is taking a vitamin D supplement, which comes from a natural source: cod liver oil.

Fruits and Veggies: The More You Eat, the More You Lose!

You don't have to be a vegetarian, but you don't ever have to restrict the number of vegetables and fruits you consume. In my experience as a weight-loss specialist, I have never seen a case where someone gained weight from eating too many vegetables and fruits. In fact, research shows that the more vegetables and fruits you consume in a day, the more weight you will lose.

Eating five a day, thirty-five a week, is a must. This should be one of the top items on your to-do list. If you are not used to eating a lot of vegetables and fruits, start by adding one or two servings each day. Add an extra serving of vegetables at a meal or have a piece of fruit for a snack. The key is to keep increasing the number of vegetables and fruits you consume each day. There is no limit.

RED FOODS REDUCE THE RISK OF HEART ATTACK AND CANCER

The micronutrient lycopene provides the vibrant red color to fruits and vegetables in this category. Another beneficial micronutrient, anthocyanins, adds to the color. Anthocyanins are a type of antioxidant known as a flavonoid, one of the most potent antioxidants known. A newly discovered flavanoid, fisetin, which is found in strawberries and other foods, has been found to reduce inflammation and helps reduce the complications of diabetes.

RED VEGETABLES

- Beets
- Radishes
- Red bell peppers
- Red cabbage
- Tomatoes

RED FRUITS

- Apples
- Blood oranges
- Cherries
- Cranberries
- Guava
- Pink grapefruit
- Pomegranates
- Raspberries
- Red grapes
- Red pears
- Rhubarb
- Strawberries
- Watermelon

Red vegetables and fruits can reduce the risk of heart attacks and protect against many cancers, especially prostate cancer. Cooked tomatoes and tomato paste are very high in lycopene, but canned tomatoes, even canned organic tomatoes, can contain the endocrine-disrupting chemical BPA, transferred from the lining of the can. For more information on BPA, see chapter 8.

Jars of spaghetti sauce also have a lot of lycopene, but most brands also contain a lot of sugar, sodium, and chemicals. The bottom line? Jars of spaghetti sauce can be healthy (read the labels), but I recommend fresh tomatoes as the best source of lycopene without getting all the sodium, preservatives, and other chemicals.

The Red Vitamin, B_{12}, Is Not in Most Veggies or Fruits

Vitamin B_{12} is a red-colored vitamin. If you have ever had an injection of vitamin B_{12}, you may have noticed its bright red appearance. Vitamin B_{12} is important for the health of red blood cells, but it is missing from most vegetables and fruits. In fact, vegetarians are at high risk for vitamin B_{12} deficiency, which can lead to pernicious anemia as well as neurologic problems.

Red meat has high amounts of vitamin B_{12}. Other sources of vitamin B_{12} include fish, meat, poultry, eggs, milk, and milk products. Another way of getting enough vitamin B_{12} is to take a supplement or eat a food that has been fortified.

The usual dose of vitamin B_{12} is 500 to 1000 mcg daily. Injections of vitamin B_{12} are rarely needed. But in certain situations, the body cannot absorb vitamin B_{12} and injections or a vitamin B_{12} nasal spray is necessary.

ORANGE AND YELLOW FOODS IMPROVE EYESIGHT AND HEALING

Orange and yellow vegetables and fruits contain nutrients called carotenoids that are related to vitamin A. Carotenoids are known to enhance immune function, improve eye sight, and help in wound healing.

Limit Raw Cruciferous Vegetables

You should limit the amount of raw cruciferous vegetables you consume, such as brocolli, kale, and cabbage, to three or four servings per day. This is because excessive amounts of some types of raw cruciferous vegetables can inhibit thyroid function (see chapter 5). You can eat as many cruciferous veggies as you want, as long as they are cooked.

ORANGE AND YELLOW VEGETABLES

- Carrots
- Corn
- Orange bell peppers
- Pumpkins
- Squash
- Sweet potatoes
- Wax beans
- Yellow bell peppers
- Yellow tomatoes

ORANGE AND YELLOW FRUITS

- Apricots
- Cantaloupe
- Lemons
- Mangoes
- Nectarines
- Oranges
- Peaches
- Pears
- Pineapple

GREEN VEGETABLES HELP PREVENT CANCER

Green vegetables get their deep green color from a pigment you may have heard of called chlorophyll. Green vegetables may have other colors in them too, but the deep green color can mask other colors. Dark green leafy vegetables, such as spinach and collard greens, are especially high in antioxidants and B vitamins. Cruciferous green vegetables, such as broccoli, kale, cabbage, and brussels sprouts, have substances that can help prevent cancer.

GREEN VEGETABLES

- Artichokes
- Asparagus
- Bok choy
- Broccoli
- Brussels sprouts
- Cabbage
- Celery
- Collard greens
- Cucumbers
- Green beans
- Green bell peppers
- Green onions
- Kale
- Lettuce
- Okra
- Spinach
- Zucchini

GREEN FRUITS

- Green grapes
- Honeydew melon
- Kiwi
- Limes

BLUE, INDIGO, AND VIOLET FOODS FIGHT HEART DISEASE AND STROKE

Anthocyanins give the natural blue purple pigment to these fruits. They contain a lot of antioxidants and have evidence showing protection from heart disease, strokes, and cancer.

BLUE, INDIGO, AND VIOLET VEGETABLES

- Eggplant
- Purple bell peppers
- Purple cabbage
- Purple sweet potatoes
- Purple tomatoes

BLUE, INDIGO, AND VIOLET FRUITS

- Blackberries
- Blueberries
- Figs
- Plums
- Purple grapes

WHITE FOODS LOWER BLOOD PRESSURE AND CHOLESTEROL

For the better part of a decade, diet experts have recommended against eating white foods. Why? Think about all the processed high-carbohydrate white foods: white bread, mashed potatoes, white rice, white pasta, and so on. We associate white foods with those that have the nutrients stripped out. For processed white foods, this is exactly what is going on.

But there are some healthy white or pale-colored fruits and vegetables that should be included as part of your diet. I like to think of the whites as the clouds surrounding the rainbow. White fruits and vegetables contain nutrients that can lower blood pressure and cholesterol and reduce the risk for certain types of cancer.

Eat Blueberries for Better Memory

Blueberries have been shown in studies to improve cognition and reverse memory loss. They are ultrahigh in beneficial micronutrients.

Stay Away from Dried Fruit and Fruit Juice

Although packed with healthy chemicals, dried fruit and fruit juice are considered processed foods, and are very high in sugar and calories.

WHITE FOODS

- Bananas
- Cauliflower
- Corn
- Garlic
- Mushrooms
- Onions

How Micronutrient Deficiency Leads to Cravings

If your body is missing a micronutrient, vitamin, mineral, or other nutrient, the symptom may be a craving. Sometimes you crave foods that contain the missing nutrient, but sometimes you may just have a craving for a particular or unusual food. The craving persists even if you eat the food, because you aren't replacing the missing micronutrient.

It is hard to test for micronutrient deficiencies because many are found in trace amounts and there aren't even blood tests for them. A good rule of thumb is that if you consume less than thirty-five servings of vegetables and fruits each week, there is a good chance you have a micronutrient deficiency. Even if you take a vitamin pill, if you don't eat enough vegetables and fruits, there is still a chance that you could develop a craving-causing micronutrient deficiency.

Fruits and vegetables are nutrient-dense. Calorie-dense foods, on the other hand, have a lot of calories but not that many nutrients. Calorie-dense foods include high-fat foods and high-sugar foods, such as fast food, snack foods, candy, and baked goods. These foods fill your body with empty calories, missing the micronutrients you need to prevent cravings. The result is that you gain weight and your appetite is never satisfied. Your body is missing nutrients, vitamins, and minerals, and it responds with hunger and cravings.

You don't have to worry about all the different types of vitamins and minerals that you need to eat to satisfy each type of craving. If you eat all the colors of the rainbow on a consistent basis, you will be assured that you are getting enough of the micronutrients you need to prevent your "craving control center" from going whacky. By flooding the body with the nutrients contained in all the colors of the rainbow (and the clouds), the brain and body don't sense that something is missing. The brain stops sending out craving signals and the appetite quiets down to normal levels.

Avoid Sugars and Processed Carbohydrates

To beat carbohydrate and sugar cravings, you should avoid eating sugars and processed carbohydrates. Most of the carbohydrates in your diet should be the slow carbohydrates that I recommend in chapter 5, such as vegetables, fruits, whole grains with lots of fiber, and low-fat dairy products.

All carbohydrates are eventually broken down into sugar, either by the manufacturing process or by the chemicals in your body known as enzymes. Processing them means they are essentially predigested, chemically broken down into easy-to-digest particles that, once consumed, are rapidly absorbed into the bloodstream. The more processed the carbohydrate, the more rapidly it is broken down and absorbed. This leads to blood sugar spikes and insulin surges.

Poster Child for a Bad Carbohydrate

High-fructose corn syrup is one of the worst processed carbohydrates. HFCS, as it is known by most, has been maligned by just about every diet expert because of its link to obesity, diabetes, and metabolic syndrome. In fact, the corn industry is so concerned that HFCS has a bad name that they are trying to change the name to "corn sugar." HFCS is the number one sweetener used in soft drinks and other sweetened products. It is a major source of calories for many people. And on top of all that, HFCS is a fake food, which I discuss below.

SOME DISCIPLINE IS IN ORDER

Eating sugars and processed carbohydrates to quiet a carbohydrate craving is like giving a bratty child a lollipop to shut him up. It will work for a little while, but as soon as the treat is gone, the behavior returns with a vengeance. If the parent focuses on better parenting instead of giving in with a lollipop, the child's behavior will eventually become much better, making the job easier in the long run.

The Hard-to-Pronounce Ingredients in Fake Foods

Unfortunately, consumption of fake foods is on the rise, and these foods are displacing nutritious foods in our diet. It's important to read the label. If there are a lot of complicated sounding names in the ingredients, this is a food you should avoid or eat in very limited quantities. Also, watch out for the word *enriched*. This means that vitamins have been added to the food.

Frequently, manufacturers enrich unhealthy foods by adding vitamins and minerals to make them appear healthy, including breakfast cereals or margarine. Some of my patients have told me that they perceived these foods to be healthier until they started reading the ingredients list.

The same is true for carbohydrate and sugar cravings. If you give in to the craving, you will get a short-term relief: a brief feeling of calmness as your serotonin takes over (see chapter 3). But this relief is short lived and sets you up for feeling tired and washed out, later feeling anxious and having more carb cravings. This surge and spike cycle is a major cause of carbohydrate cravings. Breaking the cycle is not easy, but like good parenting, is necessary for you to beat carbohydrate cravings now and forever.

When you have a carbohydrate craving, don't eat processed carbohydrates or sugar. Try eating a healthy, hearty bowl of soup, some fruit with low-fat cheese, a hard-boiled egg, or a few ounces of cooked chicken breast. See chapter 5 for more things you can eat when you have a carbohydrate craving.

Don't Eat Fake Food

I am not talking about wax fruit. It's critical to minimize your consumption of processed food, food high in preservatives or other chemicals, artificial sweeteners, fat substitutes, and artificial colors.

As I discuss in chapter 8, in today's world, it is almost impossible to live a life devoid of all chemicals. But there is a lot you can do to reduce the amount of fake foods you consume. Become more aware of the foods you eat; read the labels and consider healthier natural alternatives. I encourage you to try new things, exploring more natural alternatives to the fake foods you are currently eating.

A LITTLE GOODNESS GOES A LONG WAY

When you do eat fake foods, do so sparingly. Don't just pile it on because it is promoted as a healthier version of the real thing. It's better to use a small amount of the real thing than a lot of the imitation. For example, use a tiny amount of butter instead of a larger amount of margarine.

FAKE FOODS

- Margarine
- Artificial sweeteners
- Fat substitutes
- Artificial colors
- Foods with a lot of preservatives or artificial coloring
- Chips and crackers (trans fat snack foods)
- Commercially baked cookies, cakes, and pies
- High-fructose corn syrup

BANISH FAKE FOODS FOR LONG-TERM SUCCESS

For many people, eliminating (or even reducing) the fake food you eat can be the most important thing you do to heal dysfunctional hunger hormones. Eliminating fake foods can make the difference between having temporary and permanent weight loss. Fake foods boost appetite and cause cravings, often for the real version of that food. Fake foods don't trigger your "stop eating" hormones to quell hunger. Fake foods backfire and cause you to eat more, not less.

Restore Gut Microflora with Yogurt

Eating a lot of fake foods can change the types of bacteria that live in your gut, known as your gut microflora. If the bacteria in your gut are not healthy, you can feel sick and tired or have a host of gastrointestinal complaints, such as bloating, diarrhea, constipation, or abdominal discomfort.

If you have been eating a lot of fake foods, take an over-the-counter probiotic, or just eat some yogurt to help restore your gut microflora to a healthy balance. Once you eliminate fake foods from your diet, your gut microflora should stay healthy without the need for long-term use of probiotics. However, I do recommend eating yogurt two or three times each week so you get new healthy bacteria from yogurt on a regular basis.

Which One Is Healthier?

Bacon bits	Real bacon
Turkey bacon	Real bacon
Soy meat substitute	Chicken breast
Fruit roll-up	Fruit
Veggie chips	Vegetables
Energy bar	Whole-grain cereal
Pancake syrup	Real maple syrup
Margarine	Butter
Processed cheese food	Real cheese
Nondairy whipped topping	Whipped cream
Diet soda	Water

Answer: The real version is always the healthier version. (Even for unhealthy foods.)

The chemicals in fake foods can sometimes cause a host of symptoms in addition to hunger and cravings, including fatigue, brain fog, depression, mood swings, headaches, bloating, and insomnia. Many of my patients tell me that these symptoms get better when they quit eating fake foods. Other patients have told me that when they stopped eating fake foods, they felt like they regained their sense of taste and smell. This in turn enabled them to enjoy their food more and feel more satisfied eating less food.

DON'T BE FOOLED BY HEALTHY NAMES

Nutrition experts have criticized a whole host of fake foods. Does anyone really believe that cheese puffs are healthy to eat? Even if a product—other than cheese puffs—is made with the intent of being healthier than the actual product, it is actually less so due to the chemical processing.

Turkey bacon can have just as many calories and fat as real bacon, and contains processed meat and lots of chemicals, including mechanically separated turkey, sodium lactate, sodium diacetate, sodium phosphates, smoke flavor, sodium erythorbate, autolyzed yeast extract, and sodium nitrite. Have you ever looked at a piece of turkey bacon? What is that strip of white that is supposed to look like the fatty part of the bacon? Turkey bacon, while it may sound good on paper, is not a healthy food.

Bacon bits contain textured soy flour, partially hydrogenated soybean oil, artificial flavors and colors, and autolyzed yeast. I do not consider bacon bits a healthy food. Real bacon is not the healthiest food you can eat, but it is a healthier choice than the imposters.

Fake meat is not healthier than a lean cut of meat. Consider a soy-based meat substitute versus lean chicken breast or a lean cut of beef or bison. The ingredients of the soy fake meat include texturized soy protein, sodium caseinate, cellulose gum, modified potato starch, autolyzed yeast extract, hydrolyzed vegetable protein, artificial flavors, maltodextrin, caramel color, and guar and xanthan gums.

Artificial sweeteners and the fat substitute olestra increase hunger and cravings because they confuse the brain by sending an inconsistent message. The brain thinks it is getting sugar or fat, but the calories never come. Hunger hormones await a nutritional event that never occurs, which stimulates cravings for the actual food. They also alter types of normal healthy bacteria that are supposed to live in our gut.

Add a Morning Snack to Beat Afternoon and Evening Cravings

Adding a high-volume snack around 10 or 11 a.m. can reduce hunger and cravings in the afternoon. For many people, a big breakfast replaces the need for a morning snack. But if you are having cravings in the afternoon or in the evenings, then adding a morning snack in addition to a big breakfast can help direct your hunger hormones in the right direction at the time that you need them.

The morning snack should be planned in advance, and you need to eat it even if you don't feel hungry. In fact, you need to make an extra effort to remind yourself to have this snack, because it may not feel natural and you won't be thinking about it at a time when you are likely to be busy at work.

Check the First Ingredient in Wheat Bread

Fake wheat bread is essentially white bread colored brown. Fake wheat bread lists "enriched wheat flour" as the first ingredient. The manufacturers may try to trick you into thinking this bread is whole wheat by adding processed fiber to increase the number of grams of dietary fiber listed and add flecks of brown color to the bread. Doesn't it seem strange to start with highly processed flour and then add back processed fiber? Fake wheat bread is the epitome of a fake food!

Look for bread that lists "whole wheat flour" as the main ingredient. Each slice should have at least 2 grams of fiber, but the best whole-wheat bread has 5 to 6 grams of fiber per slice.

Be sure to eat a healthy morning snack that contains high-volume, low-calorie foods, which I call low-caloric density foods, as discussed in chapter 6. This snack should contain slow carbohydrates. Fruits and vegetables are a great morning snack. You can also include a small amount of protein and healthy fats, but this is optional for the morning snack, because you should eat lunch at least two hours later. If you anticipate more than two hours in between the morning snack and lunch, then you should add at least 5 grams of protein.

The History of Margarine

Food scientists work to create foods that aren't what they seem. For the most part, these are unhealthy foods. Let me give you an example. Margarine was created in a laboratory to be a less expensive substitute for butter. Here are just a few of the ingredients contained in margarine: partially hydrogenated soybean oil, plant stanol esters, emulsifiers, vegetable mono- and diglycerides, soy lecithin, hydrogenated soybean oil, potassium sorbate, citric acid and calcium disodium, and artificial flavor.

For decades, doctors thought that margarine was healthy because it lacked the saturated fat found in butter that has been linked to premature atherosclerosis and cardiovascular disease, such as heart attacks and strokes. But then we discovered that margarine contains trans fat, which is even unhealthier than saturated fat. Newer margarines have been developed that claim to contain healthier fats, but even the manufacturers admit that they do contain trace amounts of unhealthy fats in addition to a whole bunch of chemicals. The research is still unclear whether these trans fat–free margarines are any healthier than butter.

STEP BY STEP

Ways to Enjoy a Healthy Morning Snack

- Choose a piece of fruit.
- Cut up some raw veggies and munch.
- Have a bowl of cereal and skim milk.
- Enjoy Greek yogurt with sliced almonds.
- Try fat-free cottage cheese and fruit.
- Eat a half turkey or ham sandwich.
- Drink a smoothie.

BEAT LATE CRAVINGS IN THE MORNING

Afternoon and evening cravings are usually caused by falling blood sugar and rising ghrelin. Eating a high-volume morning snack that contains slow carbohydrates gives your body a controlled source of energy. The morning snack also helps lower appetite-stimulating hormones and boosts appetite-suppressing hormones at the time when you need it the most.

Stave Off Salty Carb Cravings with Soup

If you have cravings for salty carbohydrates, such as chips, crackers, or pretzels, eat a bowl of healthy soup filled with lean protein, vegetables, and lots of flavor instead.

Soup gives you a lot of nutrients and a lot of volume. Make sure you use a lot of herbs and spices in your soup to add a lot of flavor. Soup is a very satisfying food, suppressing ghrelin and increasing PYY (see chapter 6). You can even add a little salt to your soup to help with the salty part of the craving. You may still crave snack foods in the beginning when you use this technique, but if you consistently eat soup instead of eating chips, crackers, or pretzels, your craving for snack foods will gradually abate.

Eat Slow Carbs Instead of Cookies, Cakes, Pies, and Pastries

Similar to the technique of using soup to stanch salty carbohydrate cravings, you can choose a sweet, slow-carbohydrate dessert or a smoothie when you have cravings for cookies, cakes, pies, or pastries, which are highly addictive. The idea is to satisfy your brain's dopamine reward system with a yummy sweet food, but one that doesn't cause blood sugar and insulin swings and helps ghrelin and PYY work to make you feel full.

ADDICTIVE FOODS SATISFY DOPAMINE

Chips, crackers, and pretzels are among the most addictive foods we know of. Many of their addictive properties involve the brain hormone dopamine, which I discuss in chapter 3. A dysfunctional dopamine system is thought to be responsible for food addiction and compulsive overeating in addition to alcoholism and drug addiction.

When you have a craving for salty carbohydrates, your body is telling you that it needs a "drug" in the form of a snack food. This type of craving is not biological in nature, but more like a craving for a drug or alcohol. Giving in to a craving for snack foods will give you short-term relief and comfort, but it only feeds the addiction, making your next craving even more intense.

Prepare for Premenstrual Cravings

For many women, premenstrual cravings are impossible to avoid. You are going to have them, no matter what—but there are ways you can avoid overeating when you have these cravings. The most common foods that women crave with PMS are chocolate and sweets.

Eat dark chocolate when you have chocolate cravings or just before you expect to have these cravings. Some of my patients have told me that eating dark chocolate not only satisfies their chocolate cravings, but they also stop having cravings for sweets and crunchy snack foods, such as chips, pretzels, or popcorn.

THE WONDERFUL PROPERTIES OF CHOCOLATE

Dark chocolate is full of antioxidants and other healthy compounds. Many of the healthy compounds in chocolate are the same as those found in the dark-colored vegetables and fruits. Chocolate causes your body to release natural painkillers known as endorphins. Chocolate contains theobromine, which has a natural stimulant and appetite suppressant. Chocolate also contains compounds that simulate the feeling of being in love. Chocolate contains natural compounds that calm anxiety and reduce depression.

SATISFY FEMALE HORMONES

PMS cravings can be very intense. Eating dark chocolate before or during cravings floods the body with the flavor of chocolate combined with powerful compounds that alleviate many of the symptoms of PMS. It allows you to satisfy your craving and feel better without overeating.

To attack cravings for sweets during PMS, you may eat a very small amount of the sweet food that you are craving (less than 100 calories) combined with a healthier food, such as fruit. Although I always recommend not giving in to carbohydrate cravings, I have found that some women have particularly strong cravings for sweets during PMS.

My usual advice for these cravings doesn't always work because the craving is driven by female hormones, including progesterone and estrogen, instead of the usual culprit, insulin. By eating a small amount of the food you crave and combining it with a healthy food, you can satisfy your PMS craving without doing major damage to your endocrine system and your waistline.

Not for Women Only

PMS is not for women only. Many of my male patients tell me they have cravings for the same foods as their wives and girlfriends when they have PMS. They may not even be aware that their significant other is having PMS at the time. Many women fill the house with chocolate, candy, chips, or desserts when they are PMS-ing. Their spouses and boyfriends crave these foods because they see them and eat more of these foods because they are there. Be aware of your significant other's menstrual calendar and understand why these foods may make an appearance in your home during certain times of the month.

You Can Eat Dark Chocolate Every Day

Everyone knows that dark chocolate is a healthy food. The unhealthy part of chocolate is the sugar and fat that is added to make it taste sweet and creamy. Many nutrition experts recommend eating a few small squares of dark chocolate every day. Eat chocolate that contains 65 percent cocoa or higher. The higher the percentage of cocoa, the healthier the chocolate. Stay away from chocolate that contains any fat other than cocoa butter. Don't eat milk chocolate or white chocolate. Avoid chocolate with fillings, although dark chocolate–covered nuts are okay from time to time.

Exercise in the Morning or at Lunchtime to Beat Late-Day Cravings

Afternoon and evening cravings can be reduced by getting some exercise earlier in the day. Many people wait until after they finish work to exercise. By the end of the day, they don't feel like exercising and usually feel hungry or have cravings at the time they planned to exercise.

Studies have shown that exercise reduces appetite, especially for three to four hours after your activity. When you exercise early in the day, the effect persists longer. Most of my patients who have afternoon hunger or cravings in the afternoon have benefited from this technique.

Will Exercise Make You Hungrier?

The answer is no; exercise will not make you hungrier. Over the years, many of my patients have told me that they are afraid to exercise because they think it will make them overeat. I guarantee this will not happen. Studies in animals have shown that increasing the amount of physical activity they get does not translate to them eating more food.

If you feel hungrier when you exercise, it may not be genuine hunger, but a smoke screen from dysfunctional hunger hormones to prevent you from losing weight. It may be that your brain appetite switch is turned on when it should be off. If you do feel hungrier when you exercise, keep eating the foods I recommend in this book. You will find that with time your appetite will adjust to your new, more active lifestyle.

Improve the Duration and Quality of Your Sleep

As I discuss in chapter 10, it is vital that you have high-quality sleep. When it comes to cravings, sleep is no exception. In fact, a lot of sleep research today is directed at understanding why sleep deprivation causes cravings, especially for high-sugar and high-carbohydrate foods. It is thought that sleep deprivation prevents sugar from properly entering brain cells, causing them to make you crave more sugar.

Having healthy sleep is like having a healthy diet. It takes hard work and doesn't always come naturally. But like all the items in the Action Plans in this book, it isn't an all-or-nothing undertaking. Practicing just a few behaviors of what we call "sleep hygiene" can get your biological clock synchronized, resulting in fewer cravings and a decreased appetite. Avoiding caffeine after noon, going to bed earlier, establishing a bedtime ritual, and making your bedroom a peaceful place are a few things you can do right now to improve your sleep.

Create a Diversion

When all else fails, if you have an intense craving for a particular food, a useful technique can be to create a diversion. Do anything you can not to give in to the craving. The idea is to take your mind off food. This technique only works if you take care of your body's biological needs. This means that you must eat a healthy balanced diet and follow all the advice of this chapter. If you are eating according to this plan and your body is not missing a nutrient, then the craving is probably a psychological addiction and not a physiologic or biologic need. Feeding this type of craving will only intensify the craving and make the habit harder to break. Use nonfood diversions to take your mind off the food you are craving.

USE THE SENSE OF SMELL TO CHANGE YOUR THINKING

Smelling a particular food item can trigger a craving for that food. The hungrier you are, the stronger your sense of smell. Retailers take advantage of this at shopping malls and at airports by pumping out tempting smells of fattening treats for sale.

Smell is an integral part of eating and has been shown in studies to have an impact on hunger hormones, primarily ghrelin. Researchers have found that hunger can enhance our ability to smell as a mechanism to help us seek out food. Researchers at the University of Cincinnati found ghrelin not only binds to traditional appetite centers of the brain but also to the olfactory bulb (the smell center) in the brain, indicating that ghrelin helps tie in our sense of smell with our appetite.

Thanks to ghrelin, the hungrier you are, the keener your sense of smell. Create a smell diversion by avoiding trigger smells and using other smells to divert your attention.

STEP BY STEP

Ways to Divert Your Attention from a Craving

- Take a shower or bath.
- Clean the toilet.
- Go for a drive.
- Exercise.
- Go outside and look at the clouds for two minutes.
- Light a candle.
- Write a letter.
- Write in a journal.
- Make a telephone call.
- Send an email to a friend or family member.
- Organize your computer files or photos.
- Draw a picture.
- Change your clothes.
- Read a book.
- Watch a movie.
- Wash your car.
- Smell eucalyptus or Vicks VapoRub.
- Internet search "complications of obesity."

Repair Faulty Metabolism

We tend to equate a slow metabolism to simply getting older; studies have shown that metabolic rate decreases a few percentage points with each passing decade. However, studies also show that having a normal metabolism is more closely linked to having healthy hormones than with age. Some people are able to maintain their youthful metabolism as they get older. They have learned to keep their metabolic hormones in balance.

Even though you can't stop getting older, there is a lot you can do to rejuvenate your metabolism and stop overeating. Metabolic problems often require treatment by a qualified physician. In addition to that, the Action Plan in this chapter will get your metabolism cranked up to help you lose weight and keep it off.

Plumpy Paradox Revealed

People with a slow metabolism gain weight or have difficulty losing weight even though they eat healthy foods and exercise regularly. Most people with a weight problem have a metabolism that is slower than it should be. Even a very tiny decrease in your metabolic rate will result in a slow but steady weight gain over time. The average woman burns 9 to 10 calories per pound per day, and the average man burns 10 to 11 calories per pound per day.

***action*plan**

Fix a Faulty Metabolism

- *Eat slow carbohydrates.*
- *Combine protein with carbohydrates.*
- *Have a sweet, slow-carbohydrate dessert.*
- *Eat low-fat dairy products.*
- *Eat less fat.*
- *Spice it up!*
- *Eat for your thyroid.*
- *Build muscle.*
- *Be prepared.*
- *Exercise.*
- *Turn down the thermostat.*
- *Get the right micronutrients.*

Even a 1 to 2 percent decrease in your metabolic rate can result in gaining weight without any changes in your diet or exercise routine. Small hormonal changes can cause your metabolism to slow down, and once it starts slowing down, you're more prone to gaining weight.

I've heard the story from my patients so many times: Without any changes in their eating or exercise routine, they started gaining weight. The weight just came from nowhere. I typically perform a full medical evaluation to rule out other causes of weight gain, but for the vast majority of my patients, the diagnosis is a slow metabolism. What once worked for them is no longer working.

BEGIN BY LEARNING ABOUT YOUR METABOLIC HORMONES

To fix a faulty metabolism, you need to understand your metabolic hormones, how they might be off track, and what you can do to get them back on track and working properly. When you flip the metabolism switch, it helps you shed pounds instead of holding on to them.

The main hormones responsible for controlling your body's metabolism are insulin, thyroid hormone, testosterone, and cortisol. Doctors have known about these hormones for more than a century, but we are still learning about how they work in harmony to regulate your metabolism.

Metabolic Hormones

Insulin | Thyroid hormone | Testosterone | Cortisol

Insulin Moves Sugar into Cells for Fuel

The job of insulin is to send a message to the cells in your brain and body to take in sugar from the bloodstream and burn it as fuel. The higher your blood sugar, the more insulin your body makes. Insulin is necessary for getting the sugar into cells; without it, your cells would starve.

Food that is high in sugar or processed carbohydrates can cause a blood sugar spike, which is then followed by an insulin surge. This typically results in feelings of hunger and tiredness a few hours after eating high-sugar foods. If a food contains a slowly digested carbohydrate, as fruits and veggies do, the body has time to release insulin slowly to handle the carbohydrate in a calm and controlled manner.

THE VICIOUS CYCLE OF INSULIN RESISTANCE

The most common problem with insulin is a condition known as insulin resistance, which occurs when the body's cells stop listening to the hormone's signals. Cells don't soak up as much sugar from the bloodstream, and subsequently don't burn as much sugar for energy. Your metabolism slows and you feel tired and hungry.

If you've got insulin resistance, there is a really good chance you have leptin resistance too. When this happens, the body accumulates fat in the midsection. Once you start gaining weight, your body responds by increasing the amount of body fat. Leptin resistance makes the body reset its set point so that overweight feels normal, a serious problem I discuss in chapter 7.

The effects of insulin resistance set up a vicious cycle causing even more insulin resistance. Your body is making huge amounts of insulin, but your cells are not listening to its signals. As a result, you feel very hungry and particularly crave sugar. Your cells mistakenly think that eating sugar will solve the problem, but the problem is resistance in your cells.

Insulin resistance damages the mitochondria of muscle cells, which are responsible for producing energy and burning fuel. Insulin resistance causes fat cells to release excess amounts of blood fats, known as triglycerides, and free fatty acids. The liver accumulates fat, which leads to more insulin resistance. These substances interfere with the proper functioning of many hormones, including insulin itself. Insulin resistance also causes problems in the brain; fullness signals can't get through.

Do You Have Insulin Resistance?

___ Do you crave sugary or starchy foods?
___ Do you experience low blood sugar an hour or two after eating?
___ Is your metabolism slow?
___ Do you have skin tags (tiny flaps usually on the neck or armpits)?
___ Do you have a dark velvety rash around your neck or under your arms?

___ Is your waistline more than 35 inches (89 cm) (women) or 40 inches (102 cm) (men)?

___ Do you exercise less than two hours per week?

___ Have you given birth to a baby more than 9 pounds (4 kg)?

___ Do you frequently feel tired?

___ Is your blood pressure more than 140/90 or do you take blood pressure medications?

___ Is your HDL "good" cholesterol less than 45 mg/dL (women) or less than 35 mg/dL (men)?

___ Is your triglyceride level more than 150 mg/dL?

___ Is your fasting blood sugar more than 95 mg/dL?

___ Have you been told you have metabolic syndrome?

___ Do you have a fatty liver?

___ Do you have cardiovascular disease?

___ Do you have a parent or sibling with diabetes, cardiovascular disease, or high blood pressure?

If you answered yes to any of these questions, there is a strong chance you have insulin resistance. The more yes answers you have, the greater your chances of having insulin resistance.

STEP BY STEP

Ways to Combat Insulin Resistance

- Normalize your body weight.
- Eat a balanced diet.
- Exercise every day.
- Get enough good-quality sleep.

Thyroid Hormone Regulates Metabolism, Body Temperature, Memory, and Mood

The thyroid hormone is responsible for a vast number of bodily functions, most important metabolism. Thyroid problems are very common, especially among women, and are responsible for metabolic dysfunction in as many as 27 million Americans. Half of those don't even know they have a problem.

Thyroid hormone regulates your body temperature by controlling the rate you burn calories. Thyroid hormone also regulates the speed of your heart and bowels, as well as your memory and mood. When the thyroid becomes underactive, a condition known as hypothyroidism, your metabolism slows and you feel tired and gain weight.

Is Your Thyroid Hormone Down?

___ Are you gaining weight without any change in diet or exercise?
___ Do you feel tired?
___ Do you feel cold?
___ Do you have dry skin?
___ Are your fingernails brittle?
___ Are you constipated?
___ Do you have muscle aches or cramps?
___ Do you feel depressed?
___ Is your hair shedding?
___ Do you have a swelling in the front of your neck?
___ Are your legs swelling?
___ Do you have high cholesterol?
___ Is your heart beating slowly?
___ Have you noticed an increase in allergy symptoms?
___ Is your voice hoarse?

If you have any of these symptoms, you should see your doctor to get checked for hypothyroidism. Just having the symptoms doesn't guarantee a diagnosis, so blood tests are needed to confirm it. And even if your thyroid tests are normal, there is a lot you can do to help your thyroid function better, such as avoiding raw goitrogens (see below). Please read my book *Hormonal Balance* for more information about your thyroid.

Testosterone Makes Muscle, Which Burns Fat

Testosterone is traditionally thought of as a men's hormone, but it is not just for men. Testosterone is responsible for normal muscle growth and functioning. It is known as an anabolic hormone, meaning it builds up muscle. The more muscle you have, the higher your metabolism and the more calories your body burns. Testosterone is produced by the testicles and ovaries, as well as the adrenal glands.

If you have metabolic problems, there is a good chance your testosterone is out of balance. Both men and women experience testosterone problems, but in different ways. Insulin resistance causes men to have low testosterone and women to have high testosterone. Too high or too low, the end result is the same: Weight gain, fat gain, less muscle, and lower metabolism all result from testosterone imbalances. If you have the symptoms of testosterone imbalance, see your doctor and ask to be tested.

Men: Do You Have "Low T"?

___ Is your sex drive down?
___ Do you have erectile dysfunction?
___ Do you feel tired?
___ Do you feel depressed?
___ Have you had decreased enjoyment of life?
___ Are you shaving less frequently or have you lost body hair?
___ Are your breasts enlarged?
___ Are your testicles shrinking?
___ Have you been told that you have a low sperm count?
___ Do you have excessive sweating or hot flashes?
___ Do you have decreased muscle mass or muscle strength?
___ Are you gaining body fat?
___ Do you use tobacco or marijuana?
___ Have you noticed deterioration in work performance or your ability to play sports?
___ Do you have poor concentration or poor memory?
___ Do you have high blood pressure, diabetes, high cholesterol, or chronic obstructive pulmonary disease?
___ Do you take narcotic pain medications?

If you have any of these symptoms, see your doctor to get tested for low testosterone.

Women: Are You "High T"?

___ Do you have irregular menstrual cycles?
___ Do you have fewer than nine menstrual cycles per year?
___ Have you struggled with infertility?
___ Do you have facial hair?
___ Do you have acne or oily skin?
___ Are you losing hair, or do you have bald patches?
___ Do you have excess belly fat?
___ Do you have elevated blood sugar, prediabetes, or diabetes?
___ Do you have high blood pressure?
___ Do you have cysts in your ovaries?
___ Do you feel depressed or have mood swings?
___ Do you have terrible PMS?
___ Do you have sleep apnea?
___ Do you have a parent or a sibling with diabetes?

If you have any of these symptoms, see your doctor to get tested for high testosterone.

STEP BY STEP

Ways to Raise or Lower Testosterone

- Normalize your body weight.
- Exercise every day.
- Build muscle.
- See your doctor: Medications are often necessary. (For more information on medical treatments, please read my book *Hormonal Balance: How to Lose Weight by Understanding Your Hormones and Metabolism* [third edition].)

Cortisol Is Often Produced by Stress

Cortisol is produced by the adrenal gland and is known as a hormone primarily associated with stress. Excess cortisol raises blood pressure and blood sugar and contributes to insulin resistance. It causes weight gain, especially in the midsection, and breaks down muscle tissue, resulting in muscle loss and a lower metabolism.

Do You Have High Cortisol?

___ Are you gaining weight without any change in diet or exercise?
___ Are you gaining weight in the midsection?
___ Do you feel tired?
___ Does your skin bruise easily or do you have thin skin?
___ Do you have pink, red, or purple stretch marks?
___ Have you been told you have osteoporosis or osteopenia?
___ Are you sleeping poorly?
___ Is your sex drive down?
___ Do you have muscle weakness?
___ Do you feel anxious or depressed?
___ Is your face round?
___ Is your face red?
___ Do you have severe cystic acne?
___ Do you have a fatty hump between your shoulder blades?
___ Do you have poor memory?
___ Do you have elevated blood sugar?
___ Do you have high blood pressure?
___ Do you get frequent infections?
___ Are you under a lot of stress?
___ Do you feel amped up and fatigued at the same time (burned-out feeling)?

WARNING!

Excess Cortisol May Be Caused by Tumors

Excess cortisol can be caused by too much stress, but a more severe form of elevated cortisol can be caused by tumors of the pituitary gland or adrenal gland. If you have symptoms of excess cortisol, see your physician.

Carrots Are a Supercarb

Some nutritionists have mistakenly categorized carrots as fast carbohydrates because they have a high score on the glycemic index (GI) scale. But it turns out that carrots are one of the best carbohydrates you can eat. The high GI score is caused by a flaw in the measuring system, not a problem with carrots themselves. Carrots are packed with beta-carotene, vitamin A, vitamin C, and fiber. They are filling and crunchy and great to eat raw as a snack or cooked as part of your meal.

Eat Slow Carbohydrates

Slow carbohydrates are the healthiest type of carbohydrates. These foods take a long time to digest, and include most vegetables, fruits, nuts, seeds, legumes, whole grains, and dairy products. Slow-carbohydrate foods are sometimes referred to as "low glycemic index." A good rule of thumb is that less-processed foods are "slower" than processed foods.

Approximately 40 percent of your daily nutrition should come from eating slow carbohydrates (140 grams of carbohydrate daily, for a 1,400-calorie diet). Avoid foods with added sugar, sucrose, dextrose, maltose, fructose, honey, molasses, or high-fructose corn syrup.

White foods, such as white bread, mashed potatoes, white rice, and white pasta, are fast carbohydrates that should be eaten in limited quantities or not at all. Look for products labeled "whole grain" instead of "whole wheat." Whole-wheat bread is slower than white bread, but choose high-fiber varieties. Softer texture whole-wheat bread has processed whole-wheat flour, which can act like a fast carbohydrate.

THE DIFFERENCE BETWEEN FAST AND SLOW CARBOHYDRATES

Carbohydrates are an important part of a healthy diet. Many fad diets recommend restricting or eliminating carbohydrates—advice that results in temporary weight loss and rapid weight regain. Instead of eliminating carbohydrates, it is better to eat healthy carbohydrates, the kinds that are slowly digested, releasing sugar in a calm and controlled manner. Carbohydrates are the body's main source of energy. Your body needs a constant supply of carbohydrates in order to function properly.

Healthy, slow carbohydrates are also known as complex carbohydrates, unrefined carbohydrates, or starches. Slow carbohydrates tend to contain a lot of fiber, which helps slow digestion and the release of sugar into the bloodstream. Healthy carbohydrates also contain vitamins, minerals, and other beneficial nutrients.

Fast carbohydrates are less healthy and are known as simple carbohydrates or just plain sugar. Processed carbohydrates include refined sugar and white flour. The processing of carbohydrates replaces your body's digestive work. When you eat fast carbohydrates, sugars hit your bloodstream quickly, resulting in insulin spikes and increased hunger. Processing also removes fiber and vital nutrients, so that these foods have very little nutritional value.

SLOW CARBOHYDRATES

- Vegetables
- Fruits
- Nuts
- Seeds
- Legumes
- Whole grains
- Dairy products

Substitute Slow Carbs for Fast Carbs

FAST CARBOHYDRATES	SLOW CARBOHYDRATES
Mashed potatoes	Sweet potato
Fruit juice	Whole fruit
Instant oatmeal	Steel-cut oatmeal
White rice	Wild rice
Bread	Vegetables
Soda	Low-fat frozen yogurt
Chips	Dried edamame
Pretzels	Nuts
White pasta	Whole-grain pasta
White bread	High-fiber bread
Pasta	Beans
Grits	Corn
Sweetened low-fat yogurt	Greek yogurt

Got Sugar Cravings? Get More Sleep

Research has shown that sleep deprivation causes cravings for high-carbohydrate foods. Scientists speculate that lack of sleep causes insulin resistance in the brain, depriving it of sugar. This stimulates cravings for sweets and high-carb foods.

Take Watercress Off Your List

If you want to beat overeating, keep watercress off your shopping list. Although it is packed with antioxidants, watercress has been reported to stimulate appetite. It has been used for centuries as an herbal medicine for people who suffer from loss of appetite.

Eat More Nonstarchy Vegetables

It is better to eat more nonstarchy vegetables than starchy ones, such as potatoes, corn, lima beans, and peas. Nonstarchy vegetables are great for satisfying appetite. They are full of vitamins, minerals, fiber, and phytonutrients—and are the best source of slow carbohydrates. Nonstarchy vegetables have less than 5 grams of carbohydrate in a serving (½ cup cooked or 1 cup raw.) The more nonstarchy vegetables you eat, the better. There is no limit on this plan.

NONSTARCHY VEGETABLES

- Artichokes
- Asparagus
- Baby corn
- Bamboo shoots
- Bean sprouts
- Bok choy
- Broccoli
- Brussels sprouts
- Carrots
- Cauliflower
- Celery
- Chinese cabbage
- Collard greens
- Cucumbers
- Eggplant
- Green beans
- Green cabbage
- Hearts of palm
- Italian beans
- Kale
- Leeks
- Mushrooms
- Mustard greens
- Okra
- Onions
- Pea pods
- Peppers
- Purple cabbage
- Radishes
- Salad greens* (chicory, endive, escarole, romaine, spinach, arugula, radicchio, dandelion)
- Sprouts
- Squash (summer, zucchini)
- Sugar snap peas
- Swiss chard
- Tomatoes
- Turnip greens
- Turnips
- Wax beans

* A serving of salad greens is 2 cups (110 g)

Do You Have Hypoglycemia?

What many people know as "low blood sugar" is called reactive hypoglycemia, or food-induced hypoglycemia, or postprandial hypoglycemia. This occurs when fast carbohydrates are rapidly digested and release a lot of sugar into the bloodstream all at once. Insulin then surges, cells take in all the excess sugar, and blood sugar plummets.

The body needs sugar to function. When blood sugar levels drop rapidly, the following symptoms can occur:

___ Nervousness
___ Irritability
___ Sweating
___ Intense hunger
___ Sugar cravings
___ Weakness
___ Rapid heartbeat
___ Headache
___ Flushing
___ Nausea
___ Tingling in the hands or feet or both

Symptoms typically occur two to three hours after eating fast carbohydrates and may be mild or severe. The treatment for hypoglycemia is to eat slow carbohydrates instead of fast ones, eat protein, and avoid alcohol. Because of its effects on the way your body's cells function, alcohol tends to exaggerate the symptoms of hypoglycemia. Regular exercise also helps diminish the symptoms of hypoglycemia.

Eat a Salad After Dinner

A weight loss technique well known to people in France, Italy, and other European countries is to eat a salad after dinner, prior to dessert. A salad can curb your appetite and slows down eating so that antihunger hormones have a chance to kick in. Bitter salad greens such as chicory, endive, escarole, radicchio, and dandelion can be especially helpful turning off hunger.

Quinoa ("Keen-wah")

Quinoa is a protein-rich grain with a nutty flavor and crunchy texture. It is packed full of slow carbohydrates. Although quinoa is considered a grain, it is actually a relative of spinach and Swiss chard. The protein found in quinoa is complete, which means it contains all of the essential amino acids. This makes it an especially good choice for people who don't eat a lot of meat. Quinoa is a great source of manganese, magnesium, copper, iron, and phosphorus.

Frozen Berries Are Great Money Savers

Fresh berries, especially out of season, can cost an arm and a leg. But frozen strawberries, blueberries, blackberries, and raspberries are inexpensive and easy to find at most grocery stores. They are great in smoothies or thawed as a topping for yogurt or fat-free cottage cheese.

This technique is especially helpful in restaurants where you may be tempted to order a high-calorie dessert. If you eat a salad before dessert, you'll be more inclined to just have a taste of the unhealthy dessert.

Choose Whole Grains to Slow Down Your Gut

Whole grains are one of the best sources of slow carbohydrates. Whole grains are seeds from grassy plants, such as wheat, oats, barley, corn, and rice. They contain more fiber, protein, vitamins, and minerals than processed grains.

WHOLE GRAINS

- Barley
- Brown rice or wild rice
- Buckwheat (kasha)
- Bulgur
- Corn
- Couscous
- Cracked wheat
- Flaxseed
- Millet
- Oats
- Quinoa
- Spelt
- Wheatberries
- Whole rye

Choose Slow-Carb Fruits

All fruit is healthy, but I recommend eating more slow-carbohydrate fruits. You can still eat fast-carb fruits, but they should not be your only source of fruit. Try to limit these to three or four servings daily.

SLOW-CARB FRUITS

- Apples
- Apricots
- Blackberries
- Blueberries
- Cantaloupe
- Grapefruit
- Guavas
- Honeydew melon
- Kiwifruit
- Nectarines
- Oranges
- Papaya
- Peaches
- Pears
- Pineapple
- Plums
- Raspberries
- Rhubarb
- Strawberries
- Watermelon

FAST-CARB FRUITS

- Bananas
- Cherries
- Figs
- Grapes
- Mangoes
- Tangerines

Combine Protein with Carbohydrates

Combining protein and carbohydrates at meals and snacks is one of the best ways to beat overeating. That's because the combination of protein and carbs maintains stable blood sugar levels and keeps your metabolism up. Pairing carbohydrates with protein turns any carbohydrate into a slow carbohydrate, allowing sugar to enter the bloodstream slowly.

For example, if you eat a fruit and cereal, toast and jam, or any pure carbohydrate breakfast, your blood sugar will spike. In a couple of hours, you'll feel hungry and tired. But, if you add some protein, such as scrambled egg whites or a serving of fat-free cottage cheese, your blood sugar (and appetite) will remain stable. You'll feel less fatigued and have an easier time staying satisfied until lunch.

Turkey Sandwich on White Bread

You have learned that white bread is bad because it contains processed white flour. But when combined with protein, white bread behaves as a slow carbohydrate. The protein from the turkey slows digestion of the bread, reducing the impact on blood sugar. Adding lettuce and tomato to your sandwich makes it even healthier!

Don't Drink Milk if You're Trying to Lose Weight

Nutritionally, low-fat or skim milk contains a healthy combination of nutrients, but for weight loss, it is not helpful. Just like other caloric beverages, milk contains empty calories.

If you're trying to lose weight, you should not drink milk. This includes skim milk, soy milk, rice milk, almond milk, or any other kind of milk.

I recommend using a little milk in coffee, tea, or cereal, or using it in cooking. If you are worried about not getting enough calcium, you should take a calcium supplement or eat more low-fat dairy products.

Have a Sweet, Slow-Carbohydrate Dessert

Many dieters wait to splurge on a dessert every once in a while, eating very unhealthy items. Instead, you should eat a sweet, slow-carbohydrate dessert at least four nights a week. Eating a sweet dessert with slow carbohydrates has been shown to be an effective aid to weight loss.

In one study, participants who ate a sugar-free, low-fat dessert at least four times a week lost more weight than those who ate no desserts. A sweet, slow-carbohydrate dessert helps you feel full and satisfied at the end of the day. The sweet flavor helps satisfy carbohydrate cravings and the slow carbs prevent insulin and blood sugar spikes. The carbohydrates also help stimulate brain serotonin production, which improves mood and helps you have a deep restful sleep.

SWEET, SLOW-CARBOHYDRATE DESSERTS

- Cereal with fruit and skim milk or yogurt
- Low-calorie frozen yogurt
- Low-calorie frozen treats
- Fruit with angel food cake
- Smoothies
- Yogurt with muesli

Enjoy Low-fat Dairy Products

I recommend eating at least two or three servings of low-fat dairy products every day. These products contain the right blend of protein, calcium, and vitamin D to keep your metabolic hormones functioning in high gear. In addition to being low in calories, they are heavy and thick and keep you feeling full for a long time.

LOW-FAT DAIRY PRODUCTS

- Fat-free cottage cheese
- Fat-free sour cream
- Greek yogurt
- Nonfat yogurt
- Nonfat or low-fat cheese (hard cheeses)
- Fat-free cream cheese
- Low-calorie frozen desserts
- Sugar-free pudding made with skim milk

LOW-FAT DAIRY PRODUCTS (cont.)

- Smoothies
- Low-fat frozen yogurt
- Skim milk (in small amounts with cereal or in recipes)

Best Cheeses

Parmesan
Low-fat mozzarella string cheese
2 percent milk cheeses (Swiss, Cheddar, Colby)

Be Sure to Eat 30 Percent Healthy Fat

Your diet should contain 30 percent healthy fat. You have probably read a lot of diet books that have told you to eat less fat. They all this because it is true. High-fat diets slow your metabolic rate and cause cravings for more high-fat foods.

It's important to check your fat consumption from time to time because we live in such a high-fat society that keeping under the 30 percent mark can be a challenge. If you eat "normal" food, it probably has more than 30 percent fat in it.

The average American's diet contains 35 to 40 percent fat. Studies have shown that trimming just a few percentage points of fat in your diet has a dramatic effect on alleviating insulin resistance and helps you lose weight.

Spice It Up!

Many people try to make food taste better by adding butter or cream. Instead, try adding herbs and spices to your food. Adding herbs and spices can add a new dimension and help you control your appetite. When food tastes good, it is more satisfying. Spicy foods also help reduce appetite and help you feel full quicker, reducing the number of calories it takes to make you feel full.

Prepeel a Couple of Hard-boiled Eggs

Hard-boiled eggs can be eaten with just about any food to add protein and slow down the carbs. Keep a couple of peeled hard-boiled eggs in the refrigerator so they are always readily available.

Carry a Pepper Shaker "To Go"

Buy a camping gear salt shaker with a removable top, and fill it with your favorite chili powder, cayenne pepper, or paprika. Keep it in your pocket and sprinkle it on food when you are on the go.

Herbs and spices have virtually zero calories but tons of flavor. You can add herbs and spices to just about anything—meats, vegetables, soups, seafood, and salad dressing. They can change a bland dish to one packed with zest. Many herbs and spices can boost metabolism, decrease appetite, and help you burn fat.

CHILI PEPPERS BRING THE HEAT

Chili peppers boost metabolism by causing your body to generate heat. The chemical in chili peppers, capsaicin, stimulates a process known as thermogenesis: converting extra calories into heat. Habanero, cayenne, and jalapeño peppers all contain high amounts of capsaicin and are a great addition to your dishes. Paprika also contains a lot of capsaicin. I recommend adding any type of hot pepper to your meals as often as possible. Most people are able to eat more hot peppers over time, as their body gets used to the capsaicin.

POUR ON THE HOT SAUCE

Putting hot sauce on your food is a great way to spice up your food and give your metabolism a little kick at the same time. There are so many different brands of hot sauces available, and each region has local specialties. I try to buy a bottle everywhere I travel. Dash hot sauce on everything you eat—from scrambled eggs to soups and sandwiches.

HOLD THE SALT; PASS THE PEPPER

Black pepper boosts metabolism and is a natural fat burner, similar to chili peppers. A chemical in black pepper, piperine, creates the pungent taste and stimulates receptors in the brain. Researchers believe that black pepper increases the amount of energy needed to digest food, resulting in more calorie burning. Freshly ground black pepper has the most piperine, so add it generously.

MUSTARD IS FOR MORE THAN SANDWICHES

Use it in salad dressings and as a marinade for chicken, fish, or pork. Besides adding flavor, mustard helps burn fat. The spicier the mustard, the more it boosts metabolism. Asian mustard is the spiciest, but any mustard can be a tasty addition to your meals.

Mustard is the perfect substitute for mayonnaise, olive oil, or butter. It is fat-free, low in carbs, and practically calorie-free. Mustard contains omega-3 fatty acids, selenium, manganese, magnesium, niacin, and zinc.

GARLIC HAS MANY HEALTH BENEFITS

Studies have shown that garlic has many health benefits, including lowering cholesterol and blood pressure, as well as raising levels of HDL ("good") cholesterol. The pungent aroma and flavor of raw chopped or pressed garlic is a great complement to salad dressing, and can be used to flavor lean cuts of meat or seafood. Whole, baked garlic cloves have a sweet, creamy flavor and can be substituted for butter and spread on whole-grain bread. Raw or cooked, garlic's intense flavor and aroma are a great way to substitute taste for calories.

CINNAMON AIDS INSULIN AND CHOLESTEROL LEVELS

Adding just a ½ teaspoon of cinnamon to your food every day has numerous health benefits, including helping insulin function well. Studies have shown that cinnamon can lower blood sugar and cholesterol levels. Scientists speculate that cinnamon helps with weight loss because it slows the digestion of carbohydrates. Ground cinnamon can be used in recipes, or you can make a cinnamon tea using cinnamon sticks. Cinnamon can also be added to oatmeal, coffee, vegetables, or sweet potatoes, or as a flavoring for meat. The active components of cinnamon are not damaged by the cooking process.

GINGER: A WEIGHT-LOSS TOOL FOR CENTURIES

Even though there's little scientific research on the effects of ginger for weight loss, ginger has been used as such for centuries. It is thought that ginger increases calorie-burning by making cells use more energy. It can lower cholesterol and help calm an upset stomach. Drinking ginger tea and using ginger as a spice can be a great way to add this beneficial root to your diet.

TURMERIC INHIBITS FAT GROWTH

Turmeric is a common spice in Indian food that may help decrease absorption of fat by the intestines. Scientists have found that curcumin, a beneficial substance known as a polyphenol, is its active ingredient. Curcumin has been shown in animal studies to cause weight loss by inhibiting the growth of fat cells.

Too Much of a Good Thing

Be aware that cinnamon contains a chemical called coumarin, which can cause liver damage if consumed in large quantities (more than 4 teaspoons [9 g] per day).

Grow Your Own Herbs

Growing herbs is easy and fun. It's a great way to have fresh herbs around all the time. You can easily make homegrown herbs organic by avoiding pesticides and fertilizers. Keeping the fertilizer away from your herbs will result in a smaller, but more flavorful plant. You don't need much space, just a few pots and a sunny area. Plant basil, oregano, parsley, mint, or rosemary, and remember to water them a few times each week.

HEALTHFUL AND AROMATIC OREGANO

Oregano is an aromatic herb that can be used to flavor recipes such as tomato sauces, meats, and casseroles. Oregano has potent antioxidant properties and has been shown to stop the growth of inflammation-causing bacteria. Oregano contains omega-3 fatty acids, iron, manganese, calcium, vitamin C, and vitamin A.

TASTY BASIL SOOTHES AND STRENGTHENS

Basil, a flavorful addition to all types of dishes, may lower cortisol levels related to stress and can help reduce appetite and cravings. Basil is full of antioxidant compounds. It has been reported to lower blood pressure and helps boost immune system function.

ROSEMARY CALMS AND SLOWS DIGESTION

Rosemary is a fragrant herb with a citrus pine flavor. It is popular in Mediterranean dishes and is typically used to flavor meats, vegetables, and potatoes. Rosemary has been shown to enhance the breakdown of neurotransmitters in the brain, which scientists believe may be responsible for its calming effect. Rosemary contains a substance called carnosic acid, which inhibits the breakdown of dietary fat, slowing digestion and helping you feel full longer.

MINT IS A NATURAL APPETITE SUPPRESSANT

Studies have shown that dieters who consume mint on a regular basis consume fewer calories. Even smelling peppermint oil can help decrease appetite. Mint increases alertness and energy and can reduce snacking to boost energy levels. Use mint in cooking, salads, or tea.

EAT LESS SODIUM

It is best to limit salt intake to 1500 to 3000 mg daily. The main difference between table salt, kosher salt, and sea salt is the size of the granule. All types of salt contain the minerals sodium and chloride. The smaller the granule size, the more sodium is contained in a teaspoon of salt. Table salt is made up of very small crystals and contains the most sodium. Sea salt and kosher salt contain larger granules, reducing the amount of sodium overall. Light salt contains a blend of regular salt and potassium chloride.

Regardless of which type of salt you use, it is important not to get too much. One way to get less salt is to reduce the amount in your cooking and then add a small amount after the food is cooked.

Sodium in 1 Teaspoon of Salt:

Table salt:	2300 mg
Kosher salt:	1800 mg
Sea salt:	1600 mg
Light salt:	1150 mg

Eat for Your Thyroid

Even if your doctor has told you that your thyroid is functioning normally, you still need to do your part to make sure it functions at its best. Consume lots of antioxidants in foods such as fruits, vegetables, nuts, and whole grains.

PASS THE IODINE, PLEASE

Iodine is an element that is necessary for the thyroid to function normally. A hundred years ago, iodine deficiency was common, but today it is rare because iodine (in the form of potassium iodide) is added to salt. Although seafood and other foods, such as dairy products and commercially baked bread, do contain some iodine, most of the iodine that the body needs comes from iodized salt. The recommended daily allowance for iodine is 150 mcg per day, but I recommend getting closer to 500 mcg of iodine daily. The average American gets 300 to 500 mcg of iodine daily in their diet.

BEWARE OF RAW GOITROGENS

Goitrogens are found in cruciferous vegetables, such as cabbage, broccoli, brussels sprouts, turnips, rutabaga, kohlrabi, radishes, cauliflower, cassava, millet, and kale. These vegetables contain naturally occurring substances known as isothiocyanates that interfere with the function of the thyroid gland. They are only considered a problem when the food is consumed raw.

Make Your Own Spice Blend

I like to make a custom blend of dried crushed herbs, garlic powder, and black pepper. This can be used for recipes throughout the week. I try different blends— although I do have my favorites. Try garlic powder, lemon pepper, and paprika or a preblended product such as Mrs. Dash.

When Stuck on a Plateau, Check Your Thyroid

Rapid weight loss can sometimes put the body into a state of stress that causes the thyroid to stop working. Essentially, the thyroid senses that the body is starving and shuts off production of thyroid hormone to halt this perceived starvation. If you are following an ultrastrict diet and have reached a plateau, take a short break from your diet, but don't go hog wild. Then resume healthy eating following my guidelines instead of going back to the strict diet.

So-Called Iodine Allergy

Oftentimes an allergic reaction to seafood is misdiagnosed as an iodine allergy, as are allergic reactions to antiseptics that contain iodine or iodine dye used for CT scans. But doctors debate the existence of true iodine allergy. Reactions typically blamed on an allergy to iodine are usually an allergy or nonallergic reaction to a different ingredient. Everyone needs iodine. Many people who have been told they are allergic to iodine don't have a true allergy.

There's no evidence that these foods cause health problems for most people, though; in fact, they have many health benefits. The key is not to eliminate these foods, but don't eat excessive amounts of raw goitrogens .

DON'T EAT TOO MUCH SOY

Soy products are considered endocrine disruptors, although they also have many health benefits. Soy is a healthy source of protein and contains natural estrogen-like compounds. When it comes to the thyroid, however, too much soy can cause problems. Studies have shown that overconsumption of soy products block the absorption and action of thyroid hormone and may even induce autoimmune thyroid disease. (Don't worry about using Chinese soy sauce on your wild rice, though; you'd have to drink bottles before it would do harm, and the sodium would be worse.)

The estrogen-like effect of soy also increases binding proteins in the blood, lowering free thyroid hormone levels. Soy menopause products that contain isoflavones can also cause thyroid problems. It's okay to have some soy; just don't overdo it (See chapter 8).

Tip the Scales on Muscle and Body Fat

The muscle and fat balance in your body is one of the primary determinants of your metabolism. Increasing your muscle mass will boost metabolism, allowing you to burn more calories on a daily basis. It helps to focus on exercises that will help you build muscle and decrease your percentage of body fat (see chapter 9 for suggestions).

Be Prepared to Relax

The stress of everyday life has a way of creeping into our sense of well-being, raising cortisol and boosting insulin resistance. Relaxation helps lower the stress hormone cortisol and decreases insulin resistance.

When it comes to your metabolic hormones, one of the best forms of relaxation is planning. Take time whenever you can to prepare for the expected. If you know you are going to come home from work too tired to make a healthy dinner, make dinner in advance. Coming home and enjoying it will be a relaxing experience.

An underactive adrenal gland is a serious problem that can be fatal without treatment. Treatment involves taking steroid medications to replace the cortisol that the adrenal gland isn't making.

Exercise to Your Hormones' Content

For your metabolic hormones, it helps to exercise every day. Aerobic exercise helps burn calories and builds cardiopulmonary stamina. One bout of exercise raises your metabolism for up to twenty-four hours. If you exercise every day, you can keep your metabolism in this accelerated rate all the time.

Resistance or weight training helps build muscle and burn fat, another key determinant in overall metabolic rate. For more on the best way to exercise, please see chapter 9.

Check Your Adrenals if Your Salt Cravings Are Real

Many people who crave salty carbohydrates really are craving the carbohydrates and prefer foods such as chips, pretzels, and popcorn. True salt cravings, however, can be a symptom of decreased cortisol production by the adrenal glands. This is a medical problem known as Addison's disease. If you have salt cravings, see your doctor to get your adrenal glands checked.

Turn Down the Thermostat

It is good to know that when you cool your body down, it helps you lose weight. It is better not to make yourself feel cold, but a small decrease in the temperature your body is exposed to can make a big difference. Swimming, even in warm water, is especially good at drawing out body heat, forcing your body to burn more calories.

Studies of animals have shown that lowering room temperature just a couple of degrees can shift metabolic rate enough to get them to lose weight without a change in diet or exercise pattern. Cold exposure makes white fat act like metabolically active brown fat, which burns more calories. Cold also exerts an insulin-like effect on cells, causing them to take up glucose from the blood.

STEP BY STEP

Ways to Boost Thermogenesis

- Exercise in cold weather.
- Go swimming.
- Turn down the temperature.
- Drink ice water throughout the day.

Get the Right Micronutrients

Vitamins, minerals, and supplements can help metabolic hormones function optimally. As I've said throughout this book (and especially in chapter 7), antioxidants are the most important micronutrient when it comes to beating inflammation and balancing hormones. I always recommend trying to get the bulk of your micronutrients from the foods that you eat, but if your diet is lacking, here is a guide to what you need to keep metabolic hormones working properly.

DOSAGES TO BOOST YOUR METABOLISM

- Omega-3 fish oil 2000 to 4000 mg daily
- Alpha-lipoic acid 400 to 600 mg daily
- Calcium 1200 to 1500 mg daily
- Vitamin D 1000 to 3000 IU daily
- Vitamin B_6 25 to 50 mg daily
- Vitamin B_{12} 500 to 1000 mcg daily
- Vitamin E 400 IU daily
- Chromium 500 mcg daily
- Vanadium 50 mg daily
- Selenium 50 mcg daily
- Iodine 500 mcg daily

CHAPTER 6

Satisfy Your Gut

To beat overeating, people think they need to eat less food. But the real key is eating enough delicious low-calorie food to keep your gut satisfied. Instead of decreasing food portions, which will surely lead to overeating, the best way to lose weight and stop overeating is to manage hunger by eating satisfying foods that help you feel full longer.

Until recently, the role of the gut in appetite control has largely been ignored. We now know that the so-called gut hormones control satiety. They tell your brain that you have had enough to eat and help you feel full and satisfied after a meal. Researchers have developed a Satiety Index, which appears at the end of this chapter.

Discover Which Foods Are Most Satisfying

In general, bulky, high-volume foods, including vegetables, fruits, and whole grains, as well as low-fat dairy products that weigh a lot regardless of how many calories they contain, tend to be the most satisfying. Foods that are high in fiber and protein, such as lean meats, eggs, steel-cut oatmeal, lentils, and beans, also are satisfying.

Fatty foods, snack foods, and fast food, on the other hand, are not as satisfying as you might expect them to be. High-carbohydrate foods, such as bread

***action*plan**

Keep Your Gut Satisfied

- *Eat low-calorie density foods.*
- *Get enough fiber.*
- *Dilute higher calorie foods.*
- *Eat crunchy and chewy foods.*
- *Make it thick.*
- *Eat protein all day long.*
- *Drink calorie-free beverages.*
- *Eat slowly and wait for the fullness signal.*
- *Make your food look delicious.*
- *Prepare for challenging situations.*

and high-sugar yogurt, tend to be satisfying for the short term, but then leave you feeling hungrier just a few hours later.

Eat as Much as You Like

When it comes to satisfying gut hormones, rule number one is to fill up the gut. Make it a practice to eat heavy foods that are high in volume but low in calories. These foods are known as low–calorie density foods, and tend to have a lot of water in them. You can enhance satiety with low–calorie density foods because they take up a lot of space in your belly. They're also low in sugar and fat.

How Hormones Dictate Hunger and Fullness

Some foods are more satisfying than others because of the effect they have on the hormones produced by your stomach and intestines. The key to eating fewer calories while feeling full and satisfied is to understand how these hormones work.

When food enters your gut, the physical stretching caused by the food activates the gut hormones, which communicate with the brain to tell it how much food you just ate and what nutrients were in it. The hormones regulate your short-term (minute-to-minute) and long-term (hour-to-hour) appetite. Long-term appetite is also controlled by leptin, the subject of chapter 7.

FILLING FOODS

- Vegetables
- Fruits
- Legumes
- Whole grains
- High-fiber foods
- Low-fat dairy products
- Lean meats, poultry, and seafood
- Thick, healthy soups

Meet Ghrelin and PYY: The Key Gut Hormones

The stomach and intestines produce many hormones that stimulate the brain to send out signals for feeling hungry or full. Gut hormones are very complex, and are influenced by more than just food inside the digestive tract. They also respond to the anticipation of food: the sight, smell, and even verbal descriptions of food.

Cells in the stomach produce ghrelin, which mainly boosts appetite. Think of ghrelin as a "gremlin" in your stomach that makes you hungry. The small intestine and colon make the other key gut hormone, PYY (or peptide YY), which stops hunger. Ghrelin and PYY have opposing effects. To beat overeating, your goal is to keep ghrelin levels low and PYY high most of the time.

Gut motility, the speed at which the digestive tract moves, is also affected by ghrelin and PYY. Hormone communication and gut motility work together to control your sense of satiety.

STEP BY STEP

Ways to Eat Low-Calorie Density Foods

- Add berries to cereal.
- Have a salad before or after dinner.
- Try raw vegetables as a snack with fat-free ranch dressing.
- Have an extra portion of vegetables.
- Add more vegetables to dishes you love to eat.
- Sneak finely chopped or grated vegetables in eggs, meatloaf, casseroles, and pasta sauce.
- Eat an apple.
- Have a bowl of soup; add extra vegetables.
- Put lettuce, tomato, and onion on your sandwich.
- Grill zucchini, portobello mushrooms, onions, and eggplant instead of burgers and hot dogs.
- Substitute seasonings for oil in recipes and salad dressing.
- Try Greek yogurt or fat-free cottage cheese for a snack.
- Put fruit on top of yogurt or fat-free cottage cheese.
- Find low-calorie foods that you enjoy eating and eat more of them.
- Keep a tantalizing fresh fruit bowl out on the counter.
- Explore new recipes for vegetables and fruits.
- Keep cut-up vegetables in the refrigerator.
- Eat leaner cuts of meat.

GHRELIN, THE HUNGRY GREMLIN

People who are naturally thin tend to have the lowest ghrelin levels, while overweight people have the highest ghrelin levels. We don't know if people are born one way or the other, or if diet influences the amount of ghrelin we produce.

Eat Frequent Small Meals

Ghrelin levels (and appetite) are highest in the fasting state and decline after eating a meal. Levels gradually rise again, contributing to a rising appetite. The typical meal pattern of breakfast, lunch, and supper results in rising and falling ghrelin levels throughout the day—what's known as the ghrelin roller coaster.

To keep ghrelin (and appetite) low throughout the day, eat smaller and more frequent meals and snacks. This will help your gut stay satisfied and reduce the chances of overeating at any one meal.

Eat Slowly

Sage advice given to many of us as children: eat slowly. When you start eating, it takes at least 20 to 30 minutes for gut hormones to send signals about satiety. If you eat too quickly, you can overeat before they have a chance to kick in. Slowing down the gut helps you feel full and satisfied longer.

Ghrelin levels are at their highest when you haven't eaten for three or four hours, and at their lowest 20 to 30 minutes after eating a meal. When you eat three meals a day, ghrelin levels rise before each meal and fall after. This ebb and flow parallels what most people would consider a normal hunger pattern.

People who skip breakfast have a higher than normal ghrelin response, which usually leads to overeating at dinner. Eating more frequently will keep ghrelin and appetite low throughout the day. To control ghrelin, follow these guidelines:

- Have a big breakfast or a smaller breakfast with a midmorning snack (see examples in chapters 2 and 6).
- Have a healthy, balanced lunch (see chapter 2).
- Have a protein-rich afternoon snack (see chapters 2 and 9).
- Have a healthy, balanced supper (see chapters 2 and 6).
- Have a sweet, slow-carbohydrate dessert (see chapter 7).

WHY PYY KEEPS YOU SATISFIED

PYY levels drop before meals and rise after you eat. PYY acts to lower levels of the potent appetite-stimulating brain hormone NPY, or neuropeptide Y (see chapter 3 for more on NPY). PYY has a second effect to act directly on the gut to slow it down. Putting the brake on your gut helps you feel really full. Boosting PYY levels will quickly suppress appetite and increase feelings of satiety. Studies have also found that people who are overweight tend to have trouble making enough PYY; follow the Action Items in this chapter and you will be on your way to boosting PYY levels.

Recognize When Hormones Are Out of Whack

Many people overeat because their brains don't receive the right messages from their gut hormones. Poor eating habits or just bad genetics can cause this to happen to some people. The hormones lose their ability to work efficiently, so the fullness signal takes longer to kick in. For some people, gut hormones get so completely out of whack that they never feel full, no matter how much they eat.

How Satisfied Is Your Gut?

___ Do you eat until feeling uncomfortably full?
___ Do you feel unsatisfied after eating a meal?
___ Do you eat your meals quickly?
___ Do you eat huge portions?
___ Do you overeat at parties or restaurants?
___ Do you have cravings for meat?
___ Do you push your vegetables over to the side of the plate?
___ Do you feel hungrier after you start eating a meal than before you started?
___ Do you eat food out of a box?
___ Do you eat less than 25 grams of fiber each day?
___ Do you drink fruit juice or eat dried fruit instead of eating fresh fruit?

If you answered yes to any of these questions, you can get help by following the suggestions in this chapter. I'll show you how to fix your gut hormones so you can feel full and satisfied to beat overeating for life.

STEP BY STEP:

Avoid High-Calorie Foods

A good rule of thumb is to avoid foods that have more than 250 calories in a 4-ounce (115 g) portion.

Calories in a 4-ounce portion:

INSTEAD OF THIS . . .	EAT THIS . . .
Fried chicken (330 calories)	Grilled chicken breast (190 calories)
Ice cream (275 calories)	Low-fat frozen yogurt (190 calories)
Potato chips (620 calories)	Baked potato wedges (110 calories)

Drink High-volume Smoothies

Experts agree that drinking smoothies and weight-loss shakes instead of eating meals is an extremely useful weight-loss tool. You can increase the volume of your smoothie by adding extra ice and water, giving you more to drink and making you feel fuller with fewer calories.

In a study published in the *American Journal of Clinical Nutrition*, researchers gave subjects three different types of smoothies as a midmorning snack, all with equal calories but varied in the volume based on the amount of water and air whipped into the shake. Drinking the smoothies with the highest volume resulted in the subjects feeling the most satisfied. See chapter 2 for the perfect smoothie recipe.

Hooked on Food?

In its role as a chemical messenger, ghrelin sends signals to the brain, activating reward circuits similar to the way addictive drugs do. Similar to alcoholism and other addictions, obese people are thought to have a deranged reward system. This may explain why some people become addicted to food.

In research done at the University of Minnesota, ghrelin was injected into mice, which stimulated their appetite-activated brain reward centers. The investigators found that ghrelin is linked to the regulation of feeding behaviors through its interaction with the mesolimbic reward pathway, the so-called "cholinergic-dopaminergic reward link."

Research at the University of Geneva found that the higher the ghrelin levels, the stronger the drive to seek out food-induced rewards.

Scientists are looking for medications to address this problem, with a goal of developing a drug that could treat both compulsive overeating and alcoholism by restoring brain reward pathways to their normal states.

Make Sure to Get Enough Fiber

You should consume 25 to 35 grams of fiber every day. The best way to get fiber is through the foods you eat. Foods high in fiber also tend to be the most filling and best at suppressing ghrelin and raising PYY. Too much fiber can cause belly pain, bloating, gas, and diarrhea. Excess fiber can bind to vitamins and minerals, decreasing their absorption; however, this is unlikely if you keep your fiber intake less than 35 grams per day.

The main reason fiber makes you feel so full is because of its effect on your gut hormones. Fiber stretches out the stomach and tells ghrelin and PYY, "I'm full." Fiber makes you eat slower so your hormones have time to catch up, allowing you to feel satisfied after eating fewer calories.

THE TRUTH ABOUT FIBER SUPPLEMENTS

When it comes to weight loss, I am not convinced that fiber supplements have the same benefits as getting fiber from the foods you eat. Early studies suggested that fiber supplements could help with weight loss, but newer research indicates they don't do much good. One study from Spain found that a placebo caused weight loss similar to a fiber supplement.

Studies from the University of Connecticut and Tufts University showed that adding a fiber supplement to a low-calorie diet provided no additional weight loss compared to diet alone. Other studies have shown that you can lose weight by increasing fiber in natural foods that you eat. Nowadays, fiber is being added to foods, including bread, cereals, and even yogurt, so there are plenty of ways to get enough fiber in food.

STEP BY STEP

Ways to Fit in Fiber

- Eat a baked potato with the skin on.
- Substitute whole-grain pasta for white pasta.
- Add a cup of beans to pasta sauce or soup.
- Try lentils.
- Keep frozen fruit available for smoothies.
- Put high-fiber cereal on top of yogurt.
- Replace regular bread with high-fiber bread.
- Eat fresh fruit instead of dried fruit or drinking juice.
- Read the label; look for products with at least 2 to 3 grams of fiber per serving.

Dilute High-Calorie Foods

If you are going to eat a high-calorie food, the best thing you can do is eat a lower calorie food at the same time. Keep some extra vegetables around so that you can double or triple the vegetables in any recipe. Some recipes allow for experimentation, and you may need to add extra spices and flavorings. Add fruit to cereal or yogurt, or eat a fruit salad with your meal.

Drink Enough Water

It is important to drink 2 quarts (1.9 L) of water every day. If you don't drink enough water, the extra fiber can cause abdominal discomfort, cramping, bloating, and gas. If you get these symptoms, make sure you are drinking enough water. You may need to temporarily decrease your fiber consumption and then slowly increase back.

Add Vegetables to Your Pasta

The secret to making a healthy pasta dish is to use whole-grain pasta and add a lot of vegetables. A study published in the *American Journal of Clinical Nutrition* evaluated how adding different amounts of vegetables satisfied someone. They made three types of vegetable pasta:

- Pasta mixed with a lot of vegetables
- Pasta mixed with a modest amount of vegetables
- Pasta mixed with very few vegetables

Researchers found that it didn't matter which version of the pasta was served. The subjects reported feeling full regardless of which they ate. The weight of the meal mattered more. In fact, subjects who ate the pasta mixed with a lot of vegetables ate 400 calories less than those eating the higher calorie pasta.

HIGH-FIBER FOODS

- Apples
- Artichokes
- Bananas
- Beans
- Broccoli
- Carrots
- Chickpeas
- Lentils
- Okra
- Pears
- Raspberries
- Split peas
- Strawberries
- Turnip greens
- Whole-wheat pasta
- High-fiber bread
- High-fiber cereals
- High-fiber yogurt

STEP BY STEP

Ways to Dilute High-Calorie Foods

INSTEAD OF THIS . . .	EAT THIS . . .
Cheese pizza	Pizza with onions, peppers, and mushrooms
Scrambled eggs	Scrambled eggs with extra egg whites mixed in
Cheese omelet	Veggie cheese omelet
Spaghetti and marinara sauce	Spaghetti and marinara sauce with mushrooms, onions, and zucchini
Turkey sandwich	Turkey sandwich with lettuce, tomato, and sprouts
Macaroni and cheese	Macaroni and cheese with chopped cauliflower mixed in
Frozen entrée	Frozen entrée with a package of frozen vegetables
Protein shake	Protein smoothie with frozen fruit
Chocolate	Chocolate-covered strawberries
Cake	Cake with fruit

GO FOR VOLUME IN THE GUT

When it comes to satisfying gut hormones, the volume of the food is more important than caloric content. We crave higher calorie foods because they taste delicious, but neither the taste nor the calories make us feel full.

It is not realistic to totally avoid eating high-calorie foods. Doing so usually results in feelings of deprivation, and makes it difficult to sustain permanent weight loss. By diluting higher calorie foods with lower calorie foods, you can satisfy your cravings and your appetite. Even though you are eating more food, you will end up eating fewer calories over the long run.

Eat Crunchy and Chewy Foods

Crunchy and chewy foods are satisfying and should be part of your everyday diet. Many of my patients tell me that when they are on a diet, they miss eating crunchy foods. You should replace crunchy foods like chips, cookies, and popcorn with healthy crunchy foods.

These foods take a long time to eat, allowing time for the "I feel full" message to reach your brain. It can be difficult to intentionally slow down eating. Crunchy and chewy foods help make this easier.

CRUNCHY FOODS

- Roasted chickpeas or edamame
- Apple slices
- Carrot sticks
- Celery
- Zucchini
- Sliced bell peppers
- Radishes
- Turnips
- Pickles
- Jicama
- Lettuce
- Cucumbers
- Frozen grapes
- Nuts
- High-fiber breakfast cereal
- Whole-grain, low-fat crackers (such as Wasa Rye Crispbread)
- Toasted high-fiber bread
- High-fiber yogurt

Eat Your Vegetables (First!)

When you eat your meal, make a conscious effort to eat all of the vegetables on your plate before moving on to the other foods. This will help you fill up on lower calorie foods, leaving less room for the higher calorie foods. Your gut hormones won't know the difference!

How to Eat a Candy Bar

Some people I know just cannot give up eating candy bars. It is so hard to avoid the temptation because they are staring you in the face at the gas station, the grocery store, even the pharmacy. If you are someone who must eat a candy bar every so often, you must eat a piece of fruit first. This dilutes the sugar and fat in the candy bar and swells your gut, boosting PYY and suppressing ghrelin. The slow carbohydrates in fruit dilute the sugar in the candy bar, which helps mitigate blood sugar and insulin surges. Eating fruit with your candy bar will help you break the sugar craving cycle, a problem that I discuss in chapter 5.

CHEWY FOODS

- Steel-cut oatmeal
- Baked apples and pears
- Raw nuts
- Frozen sliced bananas
- Frozen strawberries
- Honeydew
- Cantaloupe
- Mushrooms
- Quinoa
- Barley
- Corn on the cob
- Wild rice
- Lean meat and poultry
- Shrimp
- Beef or turkey jerky (see chapter 2 for my healthy jerky recipe)

THICKER FOODS ARE MORE SATISFYING

Thick foods suppress ghrelin more effectively than watery versions. Thin liquids pass through the digestive system quickly and don't do much to satisfy gut hormones.

Researchers have studied the effects of thickness in a shake on hunger and satisfaction. Subjects in one study drank weight-loss shakes that varied in thickness but were nutritionally identical. When drinking the thicker shakes, the subjects reported less hunger afterward, compared to when they drank the thin shakes. The end result was that subjects consumed fewer total calories on the days when they consumed thick shakes compared to thin shakes.

Eat Protein All Day Long

You should eat protein in the morning and throughout the day. The goal is to have all your meals contain at least 20 to 30 percent protein. Although I typically don't recommend eating unbalanced meals or snacks, pure protein snacks are an exception. Protein snacks are especially helpful in preventing afternoon and evening hunger.

HOW MUCH PROTEIN SHOULD YOU EAT?

Experts recommend eating about 0.4 grams of protein for every pound you weigh. For example, if you weigh 180 pounds (82 kg), eat 72 grams of protein each day. See chapter 1 for more information.

STEP BY STEP

Choose a Protein Snack in the Afternoon

I advise eating a snack that contains 10 to 20 grams of protein around 3 or 4 p.m. every day. Your snack can have a small amount of carbohydrate or fat, but it should be primarily protein. Eating protein at this time of the day helps satisfy gut hormones and reduces appetite at dinnertime.

PROTEIN SNACKS

- Turkey or ham roll-ups
- Hard-boiled egg
- Beef or turkey jerky
- Fat-free cottage cheese with fruit
- Tuna
- Protein shake
- Lentils
- Steel-cut oatmeal
- Protein breakfast cereal
- Roasted edamame
- Pieces of precooked chicken breast

BEST SOURCES OF PROTEIN

- Beans
- Chickpeas
- Chicken and turkey breast
- Egg whites
- Fish
- Lean cuts of beef, bison, venison, pork, and lamb
- Lentils
- Lima beans
- Shellfish
- Split peas
- Tofu

High-protein Vegetable Hall of Fame

Green peas	8 grams of protein per 1-cup (150 g) serving
Asparagus	5 grams of protein per 1-cup (71 g) serving
Broccoli	5 grams of protein per 1-cup (71 g) serving
Shitake mushrooms	5 grams of protein per 1-cup (70 g) serving
Brussels sprouts	4 grams of protein per 1-cup (88 g) serving

Surprising Sources of Protein

Whole-grain oats have 6 grams of protein per 1-cup (80 g) serving; that's 1 gram more than an egg. Garlic is also a high-protein food, packing nearly 2 grams of protein in an ounce.

Make It Thick

Eat thick and chunky soups and sauces. Eat Greek yogurt, low-fat cottage cheese, mashed winter squash, and other thick foods. Modify your recipes to make foods thicker without making them higher in calories by adding puréed vegetables.

Drink Calorie-Free Beverages

Liquids with calories are empty calories because they aren't able to wake up gut hormones. Liquids slide through your digestive system unnoticed and you feel just as hungry or even hungrier. It is better to get all your calories through solid food and have calorie-free beverages.

But making all your beverages calorie free is not always easy to do. For the most part, beverages that are less than 20 calories per serving are okay. The best drink you can have is filtered cold water with lemon.

LOW-CALORIE BEVERAGES

- Water with lemon
- Sparkling water with a splash of juice (orange, grapefruit, cranberry)
- Tea (iced or hot)
- Coffee (iced or hot)
- Herbal tea
- Diet tonic water

Do Not Drink:

Soda | Fruit juice | Sweet tea | High-sugar sports drinks | Milk

USE ARTIFICIAL SWEETENERS SPARINGLY

It is better to drink beverages that don't contain artificial sweeteners. Some experts speculate that the excess sweetness of artificially sweetened beverages actually make you crave sugar and other sweet foods, such as candy and cookies. It is thought that artificial sweeteners may confuse the brain with a sweet flavor that has no calories. The sweet flavor makes the brain send out signals to the body to get ready for the sugar and calories it thinks is on the way but never come. The result is an intense sugar craving that can persist for hours or days. A good solution is to use artificial sweeteners as a way of lowering the calories of a food item. For example, if you add artificial sweetener to yogurt or oatmeal instead of regular sugar, you save the calories from the sugar but won't give an inconsistent message to the brain.

AVOID ALCOHOLIC BEVERAGES

If you are trying to stop overeating and lose weight, you should not drink alcoholic beverages. It is okay to drink on occasion if you are at your ideal weight. There are hundreds of studies that have reported the health benefits of drinking moderate amounts of alcoholic beverages. However, despite the known health benefits, alcoholic beverages also have empty calories. In fact, alcoholic beverages can stimulate your appetite.

Go Light on the Cheese

Limit the amount of cheese in your diet. Cheese is a good source of protein but is very high in fat and calories. Count it as a fat, not a protein.

Eat Slowly and Wait for the Fullness Signal

Nutrition experts agree that it is important to eat slowly and mindfully, taking the time to think about what you are eating. You should make a conscious effort to slow down your eating by sitting at a table and taking time to enjoy each bite. Savor the first few bites of food; you don't taste the later bites as much as the first few. Don't eat in front of the television or the computer. Don't eat while you are driving.

Remember that gut hormones take twenty to thirty minutes to kick in. Research has shown that when people eat quickly, their bodies restrict the release of the feel-full hormone, PYY, and boost levels of the hunger hormone, ghrelin. The faster you eat, the greater this impact on gut hormones. Studies have also shown that slow, mindful eating helps gut hormones increase feelings of satiety. It is thought that taking longer to eat and thinking about the food you eat allows the body and brain to better understand and react to the nutrients coming in.

EAT SLOWLY, BUT DON'T CHEW SLOWLY

Be sure you don't overchew your food. Overchewing food can liquefy and partially digest the food while it is still in your mouth. By the time it hits your gut, the predigested nutrients are absorbed too quickly. This can cause blood sugar and insulin surges and will point your gut hormones in the wrong direction. Chew your food at a normal pace, while taking the time to slow down your overall meal.

Beware of Peanut Butter!

Don't eat peanut butter! Ounce for ounce, peanut butter is one of the highest calorie foods you can eat. Peanut butter is a good source of protein, but if you are trying to lose weight, you should avoid it like the plague. Endocrinologists recommend eating peanut butter for their patients who are underweight and need to *gain* weight, not lose it.

Try PB2 instead. PB2 is a powdered peanut product that tastes like peanut butter, but with only a fraction of the calories and fat. It's great in smoothies and in recipes.

STEP BY STEP:

Ways to Slow Down Eating

- Choose peel-and-eat shrimp.
- Crack your own crab.
- Order a whole-fish dish at a restaurant.
- Snack on a few sunflower seeds in the shell.
- Shell your own edamame.
- Try corn on the cob instead of cut corn.
- Eat a grapefruit half.
- Eat high-fiber cereals.
- Snack on frozen green peas.
- Have a green salad after dinner.
- Eat with a small spoon or fork.
- Eat sitting down at the table.
- Drink a sip a of water between every bite.

Make Your Food Look Delicious

You should take time to make your food look appealing. No matter what it is, make it look delicious and decadent. Our gut hormones are more satisfied if we perceive the food to be more decadent. By making your food more visually appealing, the food will be more filling. Use real plates and silverware—even for frozen entrées—and never eat out of a box. I like to use garnishes on the plate, which can add visual appeal and let you sneak in a few extra vegetables and fruits.

Researchers from Yale University have determined that ghrelin is partly controlled by how yummy food appears, not the actual number of calories we are consuming. In one study, participants were given two identical milkshakes that contained 380 calories. One was labeled as a "diet" shake with 140 calories, the other was labeled an "indulgence" shake with 620 calories. Subjects had higher ghrelin levels in anticipation of drinking the indulgence shake and lower ghrelin levels after they drank it.

EDIBLE GARNISHES

- Cantaloupe or honeydew melon balls
- Carrot shavings
- Chopped green onions
- Chopped herbs
- Cilantro
- Dollop of fat-free sour cream
- Edible flowers
- Fresh ginger
- Jalapeño peppers
- Kabob of cherry tomatoes
- Kale
- Parsley
- Radish roses
- Red onion slice
- Roasted garlic
- Salsa
- Sliced lemons
- Sliced oranges
- Sliced tomato
- Strawberries
- Watermelon triangle

STEP BY STEP

Plan Ahead to Prevent Overeating

- Eat before you go to an event where food will be served.
- Have healthy, low-calorie foods thirty to forty-five minutes before you go.
- Ask the host if you can bring a dish, and always bring a healthy option.
- Avoid appetite-stimulating foods at the event.
- At parties, stand across the room from the food table.
- Limit alcohol or have nonalcoholic, calorie-free beverages or water.
- At a buffet, have small tastes of food instead of a large plate of food.
- In restaurants, ask your server to package up half of your entrée in a to-go container when your meal is brought out.
- Order a side of extra vegetables and eat it first.
- Wait to go through the buffet line until after everyone else has; when it has been picked over, it will be less tempting.
- Double your exercise on the day of the event.
- Spend time focusing on people, not food.
- Have fun and be in control of your environment!

Substitute Mushrooms for Beef

Eating mushrooms instead of beef will help you save calories and satisfy your gut hormones at the same time. Mushrooms have a chewy texture that is similar to beef. They are high in fiber and protein, B vitamins, potassium, and selenium.

In a study published in the journal *Appetite*, subjects were fed mushrooms or beef in a test lunch. The mushroom lunch was about 300 calories; the beef lunch was about 700 calories. Researchers found that despite the difference in calories, ratings of palatability, appetite, and satiety were similar with both meals.

STEP BY STEP

Ways to Save Calories and Still Feel Decadent

Making a few of these substitutions each week can help you lose 10 to 20 pounds (4.5 to 9 kg) in a year.

INSTEAD OF THIS . . .	EAT THIS . . .
Beef	Portobello mushroom
Hamburger	Turkey burger
Fried chicken	Grilled chicken
Pasta with high-calorie sauce	Pasta with low-calorie sauce and veggies
Rice	Baked potato with skin
Mayonnaise	Mustard
Butter	Fat-free sour cream
Cookies, cake, pastry	Fruit salad, low-fat frozen yogurt

Prepare for Challenging Situations

You should always make plans to eat in advance of a party or social event. Eating a meal thirty to forty-five minutes before the event will satisfy gut hormones right at the time you are most vulnerable, making it easier to prevent overeating at a challenging event. Following just a few of these suggestions can help prevent you from overeating at these events.

EAT BEFORE A PARTY TO BEAT OVEREATING THERE

This technique is helpful for challenging parties and social or business events. Have a healthy meal thirty to forty-five minutes before the event. Eat several servings of vegetables and fruits. Include a 4-ounce (115 g) portion of protein. Finish it off with a high-volume smoothie. You need to go past just feeling "not hungry," into "really full." Then head off for your event.

Even when you feel satisfied, you can still eat. Think about the last time you ate dessert. Chances are when you finished your meal you felt satisfied, but not enough to stop. But if you go beyond feeling satisfied to feeling really full, it is harder to eat anything. You may still eat at the party, but when you feel really full, your willpower is much stronger and you probably won't overeat.

The Satiety Index

The concept of satiety has become an important tool used by nutrition and weight-loss experts. Researchers have studied various foods and the effect on satiety. They have developed a satiety index, which is a tool for ranking various foods and their ability to make us feel full. How full are you likely to be after eating certain foods?

The Satiety Index was developed by Dr. Susanna Holt and her colleagues at Sydney University in Australia. It gives a numerical value to the feeling of fullness people experience after consuming a variety of foods all with the same number of calories. Dr. Holt fed volunteers a 240-calorie portion of different foods. Participants were asked to rate how full they felt during the following two hours. After the two hours, they were given a meal and the amount of food they ate was measured. At the end of the study, Dr. Holt concluded that different foods that contain an identical number of calories differ in their ability to satisfy appetite.

The standard measurement for the Satiety Index, a slice of white bread, was given the arbitrary value of 100, with other foods set in comparison to this. The most satisfying foods are the ones with the highest score. As a general rule, the more fiber, protein, and water a food contains, the higher the satiety score. Boiled potatoes had one of the highest scores. Air-popped popcorn had a high score because it takes up a lot of space in the belly for relatively few calories. High-sugar foods have low scores. Surprisingly, high-fat foods have low satiety scores. Just like other scoring systems, the Satiety Index should be used as a tool to help guide you to healthier choices, but it is not the gospel. For example, jelly beans had a high satiety score, but they are not a healthy food.

Sample Satiety Index Scores

The higher a food's Satiety Index score, the more filling it is.

BAKERY PRODUCTS		SNACKS		CEREALS	
Croissant	47	Mars candy bar	70	Muesli	100
Cake	65	Peanuts	84	Sustain	112
Doughnuts	68	Yogurt	88	Special K	116
White bread	100	Crisps (chips)	91	Cornflakes	118
Cookies	120	Ice cream	96	Honey Smacks	132
Crackers	127	Jelly beans	118	All-Bran	151
Grain bread	154	Popcorn	154	Oatmeal	209
Whole-meal bread	157				

HIGH-CARBOHYDRATE FOODS		HIGH-PROTEIN FOODS		FRUITS	
French fries	116	Lentils	133	Bananas	118
White pasta	119	Cheese	146	Grapes	162
Brown rice	132	Eggs	150	Apples	197
White rice	138	Baked beans	168	Oranges	202
Brown pasta	188	Beef	176		
Potatoes, boiled	323	Fish	225		

STAY SATISFIED BY PACKING ON THE FRUITS AND VEGGIES

To beat overeating, you need to be able to feel full and satisfied by eating healthy foods. The way to increase satiety with healthy foods is to keep ghrelin levels low and PYY levels high. You must eat high-volume, low-calorie foods, such as lean meats, vegetables, fruits, whole grains, and low-fat dairy products.

Add extra vegetables to your meals and eat extra fruit every chance you get. Make sure you get 25 to 35 grams of fiber each day and don't forget about having a protein snack in the afternoon. If you don't satisfy your gut, it is difficult to stick to a healthy eating plan for the long term. Eating healthy is easier when you don't have that unsatisfied feeling in your gut.

CHAPTER 7

Lower Your Body Weight Set Point

By reading this book, you're learning how hormones can make you feel hungry or full, and sometimes overeat. The glands that produce these hormones regulate appetite, cravings, metabolism, and body weight. Ultimately, there is an inner driving force that coordinates all of these mechanisms to keep your body at its ideal weight. Obesity experts refer to this as the "set point."

If you gain a little weight, the body speeds up your metabolism and sends a message to eat less so that you get back to your set point in a few days. If you lose a little weight, the reverse occurs, and you feel hungry. This is the normal process of body weight regulation. Your body wants to maintain a stable weight.

The problem (and solution) is that you can reset your set point. When you overeat and gain weight, after a while your body gets used to its new weight. You feel comfortable at this heavier weight. You feel hungry at normal times, when in reality your body has enough body fat stores to keep it going for days, weeks, or even months.

Once the set point has been reset, your body strives to maintain this higher weight. The reason most people regain weight after losing is because they never reset their set point. Researchers in Switzerland have demonstrated that it is possible for people to become "metabolically normal" after losing weight. The secret to getting your set point back to normal is to understand the hormone leptin.

In this chapter, I'll show you how to interrupt this complicated cycle, make your body more sensitive to leptin, and reset your set point.

How Leptin Controls Your Set Point

In the past three decades, scientists and medical doctors have developed an understanding of how our fat cells behave as an endocrine organ, producing hormones that regulate the set point. Fat cells produce many hormones, but most important, leptin. Leptin travels through the bloodstream and works in the brain to control the set point. Leptin is a long-term weight hormone (as opposed to short-term hunger hormones, such as ghrelin and PYY, discussed in chapter 6).

Leptin levels are seen to be a marker of nutritional status. Low leptin indicates low body weight; high leptin indicates high body weight. If someone is underweight, their leptin levels are low; metabolism slows, appetite increases, and the body is driven to gain weight. If someone is literally starving, their leptin is ultralow.

From an evolutionary perspective, leptin acts as a protector of our survival. Starvation and low body fat make leptin levels drop. This boosts appetite, slows metabolism, and drives motivation to seek food so we don't starve to death.

WHEN YOU'RE *REALLY* NEVER FULL

People with a rare hormone disruption known as leptin deficiency are hungry all the time and are very overweight. Their fat cells can't make leptin, so their brain never gets the signal that their body is ultrafat. They just keep gaining more and more weight.

People with leptin deficiency can take leptin injections and lose lots of weight without diet or exercise. The problem is that leptin deficiency is extremely rare. In my career, treating thousands of overweight and obese patients, I've never seen one case of leptin deficiency. I wish it were that simple.

*action*plan

Beat Leptin Resistance and Lower Your Set Point

- *Balance your diet.*
- *Eat the right amount of healthy fats.*
- *Eat a cup of veggies before 10 a.m.*
- *Move your body throughout the day.*
- *Hydrate yourself.*
- *Get enough quality sleep.*
- *Consume zinc, antioxidants, and omega-3 fatty acids.*
- *Identify and treat inflammation.*

The Big Problem: Leptin Resistance

Most people who are overweight make a lot of leptin. The problem is that it doesn't work properly. The massive amount of leptin is still insufficient for suppressing appetite, leaving people feeling hungry even when they shouldn't be, and leads to overeating. Even though their leptin levels are high, their brains don't recognize it.

This is known as leptin resistance. With leptin resistance, the brain isn't getting the message that it is time to stop eating. Leptin resistance results in the brain protecting the body from perceived starvation, even when a person is overweight. Leptin resistance lowers metabolism and increases overall appetite and cravings for high-calorie and junk foods.

Do You Have Leptin Resistance?

___ Do you feel hungry all the time?
___ Do you feel hungry at times when you shouldn't?
___ Do you have unexplained weight gain?
___ Is your weight slowly creeping up over time?
___ Do you have cravings for comfort foods, fast food, or high-calorie foods?
___ Are you not hungry for breakfast, or do you skip breakfast?
___ Do you overeat at supper?
___ Do you have excess body fat?
___ Do you have unusual eating patterns, or does your diet vary significantly from day to day?
___ Does weight loss stall after losing only 5 to 10 pounds (2.3 to 4.5 kg)?
___ Have you regained weight after losing it on a diet?
___ Do you have insulin resistance, metabolic syndrome, prediabetes, or diabetes?
___ Do you have a chronic infection, arthritis, asthma, or lupus?
___ Do you have high blood pressure or elevated cholesterol?
___ Do you have poor sleep, disrupted sleep, or short sleep?

If you answered yes to two or more of these questions, there is a good chance you have leptin resistance.

INFLAMMATION CAUSES LEPTIN RESISTANCE

Fat tissue plays another big role in this unhealthy condition: It produces powerful substances called cytokines that cause inflammation. Recently, researchers have discovered that inflammation causes leptin resistance. Indeed, the more fat you have, the more leptin you make, but also more cytokines. In the physiological battle, inflammation ends up winning, making the brain oblivious to leptin and causing leptin resistance.

It's common knowledge that inflammation causes many of the medical problems associated with obesity, such as heart attacks, strokes, high blood pressure, high cholesterol, and even insulin resistance and diabetes. But what may not be obvious is that these conditions also have the same treatment: When you beat inflammation, you will have found the way to reset your set point.

The key to beating leptin resistance is to reduce the amount of those inflammatory substances, cytokines, that your fat tissue is making. Fewer cytokines will produce less inflammation, leading to less leptin resistance. In other words, your brain will get the message that you're full. When you follow the eating plan in this book, your set point will go down incrementally until you reach your healthy weight.

STEP BY STEP

Ways to Beat Inflammation

- Keep a normal body weight.
- Eat the right amount of fat and calories for your body (see chapter 1).
- Eat healthy foods (see chapter 2).
- Drink enough water.
- Consume antioxidants and omega-3s.
- Keep your body physically fit (see chapter 9).
- Make healthy sleep a priority (see chapter 10).
- See your doctor regularly.

Leptin and Body Weight Regulation

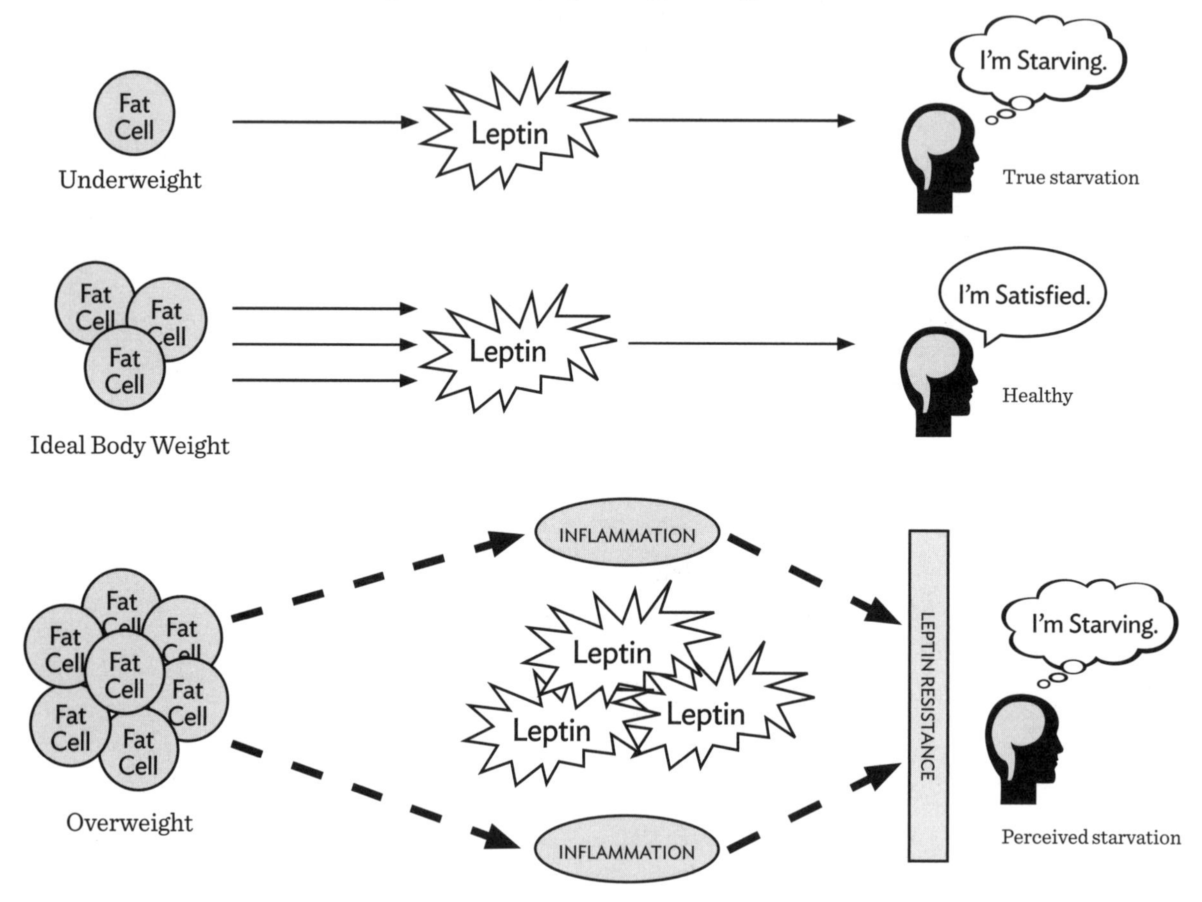

Normally, fat cells make enough leptin to give your brain accurate information about the amount of fat in your body. If body fat is normal, leptin signals the "all okay" message to maintain weight. If your body fat is low, lower leptin levels signal "starvation" to stimulate appetite and decrease metabolism. Excess fat produces inflammatory cytokines that block leptin, causing leptin resistance and resulting in "perceived starvation," inappropriate hunger, and lower metabolism despite ongoing weight gain.

With leptin resistance, there is ineffective signaling in brain appetite centers and brain motivation circuits. This leads to increased appetite, slowed metabolism, and decreased motivation to maintain healthy behaviors.

Balance Your Diet with Equal Percentages

A balanced diet means that you should eat roughly equal proportions of carbohydrates, protein, and fat every time you eat. You should also eat equal amounts of calories throughout the day, which for most people means learning to eat more in the morning and less at night.

A Balanced Meal

40 percent carbohydrate
30 percent protein
30 percent fat

WHY EATING THE WRONG SNACKS IS SO BAD

Unbalanced meals and snacks that are high in carbohydrates or high in fat don't provide the body with all the nutrients it needs. When a nutrient is missing, leptin stops working, putting the body into starvation mode. An exception to this rule is pure protein snacks, which don't have a detrimental effect on leptin.

EAT CONSISTENTLY THROUGHOUT THE DAY

Try to avoid long periods of time without eating. You should never skip meals, especially breakfast. It's best to eat at least every three or four hours while you are awake. A morning snack is optional, but if you have a long time between breakfast and lunch, then you should have a snack. If you have afternoon or evening hunger or cravings, a morning snack can be very helpful (see chapter 3).

Don't Eat High Carbohydrate Fat-Free Foods

It is logical to think that foods labeled "fat-free" are healthy. Nothing could be further from the truth. Many fat-free foods have unbalanced nutrients and tend to be high in sugar and high in calories. In fact, these high carbohydrate foods have more calories than their full-fat counterparts. Fat-free cottage cheese and other dairy products are healthy because they are high in protein.

Beat Junk Food Cravings

Eating fast food and snack foods cause the body to start craving these foods. Instead of eating junk food when you have a craving, try eating balanced meals and snacks that contain 30 percent carbohydrate, 40 percent protein, and 30 percent fat. This nutrient balance helps diminish cravings for unhealthy foods.

For example, a healthy breakfast might incorporate protein, slow carbohydrates, and a small amount of healthy fat, while a good lunch might offer lots of volume with vegetables and fruits, fiber, and protein. The key is to split the calories and make sure all three categories (carbs, protein, fat) are represented.

You should eat a substantial, balanced lunch and an afternoon snack. Unlike the morning snack, the afternoon snack is very important because most people have a longer period of time between lunch and supper. Your dinner should be light and healthy, followed by a healthy dessert. Don't listen to the old wives' tale of not eating after a certain time; the opposite is best. Eat a little all the time and never starve yourself.

What's New? The Mighty Macrophage

There is a lot of new research on fat tissue (also known as adipose tissue) and the substances produced by it. Fat tissue is composed of different types of cells. Fat cells, also known as adipocytes, are the main cell in fat tissue. But another type of cell known as the macrophage lives intermingled within the fat cells. Macrophages are white blood cells that don't just live in the bloodstream, but move into tissues throughout the body.

Macrophages live in the gut and are influenced by the food you eat. When you eat unhealthy foods, especially foods high in saturated and trans fat, macrophages become "bad," which means they cause more inflammation. Macrophages travel from the intestines to the bloodstream, where they eventually end up infiltrating fat tissue.

The macrophages that live intermingled among fat cells are known as adipose tissue macrophages, or ATMs for short. Interestingly, the ATMs are the major source of inflammation and cytokine production that has largely been attributed to fat tissue. If you eat a high-fat diet, more bad macrophages go to your fat tissue causing more inflammation and more leptin resistance.

A Balanced Day

To eat a balanced diet, you should eat roughly half your total calories by lunch, with the other half divided among the afternoon snack, supper, and dessert.

Breakfast*	30 percent of daily calories
Lunch	20 percent of daily calories
Afternoon snack	10 percent of daily calories
Supper	30 percent of daily calories
Dessert	10 percent of daily calories

Please see chapter 1 for recommended calorie intake per day.

*Calories for breakfast may be spread out for a breakfast and a morning snack.

LIFELONG CONSISTENCY IS THE GOAL

For best results, it is important to eat healthy foods consistently throughout the day as well as from day to day. You should not go on and off a diet or yo-yo diet. It is better to make permanent lifestyle changes that are sustainable for the long haul. I don't recommend eating healthy on some days and eating unhealthy on other days. Have planned rewards instead of waiting until you revolt from an ultrastrict diet, which can result in overeating and feelings of guilt.

If you go a long period of time without eating and then eat a big meal, go on and off a diet, or eat perfectly during the week and then binge on the weekends, the body becomes confused and thinks it is starving. This is both a trigger for and an indication of leptin resistance. Your brain does not know when the next meal is coming, so it sends out the signal to conserve energy. This makes you feel constantly hungry. Your metabolism slows, making you feel tired. Your body resists weight loss, and your brain tells your body to seek out high-calorie foods. If you eat consistently through the day, the body goes out of

Plan Tasty Rewards

Many dietitians will tell you that you shouldn't use food as a reward. Why not? An occasional treat can be a great way to help you stick to your long-term goals. There are so many daily temptations that total abstinence from high-calorie and high-fat foods typically results in overeating and sometimes binge eating.

Be realistic and plan to indulge yourself every so often. Decide what your reward will be and why you will get it. For example, if you eat healthy and exercise every day during the week, you will go to a favorite restaurant on Friday night. By planning the reward in advance, it gives you something to work toward and keeps you focused all week long.

starvation mode, boosting metabolism and raising energy levels. This allows you to burn off excess fat while decreasing appetite.

Eat the Right Amount of Healthy Fats

Everyone knows that eating too much fat can make you fat, but eating the wrong kind of fat also causes inflammation and leptin resistance. Eating more healthy fats and fewer unhealthy fats will help alleviate inflammation and improve the way leptin functions in the body.

Unhealthy fats contain saturated fat or trans fat and are solid at room temperature. Saturated fat comes from animal sources, such as meat, butter, and cheese, or tropical oils, such as coconut oil and palm oil. Trans fats are man-made by processing unsaturated fats and are also known as hydrogenated fats. This process creates synthetic fats that are less likely to spoil than healthier oils and are common ingredients in snack foods.

Trans fats and saturated fat cause inflammation in the body. They cause leptin resistance and make you feel hungry when you shouldn't be. Unhealthy fats are especially good at penetrating the walls of blood vessels, building up and resulting in atherosclerotic plaques, the cause of cardiovascular disease.

GET TO KNOW THE HEALTHY FATS

Many healthy foods contain both mono- and polyunsaturated fats. Monounsaturated fat, also known as MUFA, or omega-9 fatty acids, are found in fish, chicken, and vegetables. Polyunsaturated fat, also known as PUFA, is found mostly in vegetables and fish. PUFAs include both omega-3 and omega-6 fatty acids.

ENJOY THESE HEALTHY (MONOUNSATURATED AND POLYUNSATURATED) FATS

- Fish and shellfish
- Chicken and turkey breast
- Olives and olive oil
- Avocados
- Vegetable and nut oils (canola, corn, safflower, peanut, sesame)
- Nuts

- Sunflower, sesame, flax, and pumpkin seeds
- Soy products (soy oil, tofu, soy milk, tempeh)

AVOID THESE UNHEALTHY (SATURATED AND TRANS) FATS

- Fatty cuts of beef, ground beef, pork, and lamb
- Chicken skin and dark meat
- Whole-fat dairy products (milk, butter, cheese, ice cream)
- Commercially baked pastries, cakes, cookies, and muffins
- Packaged snack foods (crackers, microwave popcorn, chips)
- Margarine
- Vegetable shortening
- Fried foods
  (French fries, fried chicken, chicken nuggets, breaded fish, doughnuts)
- Candy bars
- Palm oil
- Coconut oil

WHY UNHEALTHY FATS LEAD TO CRAVINGS

Unhealthy fats, especially those found in snack foods and fast food, tend to have an addictive quality and lead to cravings for more unhealthy foods. Snack foods, especially crunchy snack foods, stimulate the brain's dopamine reward system (see chapter 3). But there can be a different cause for these cravings. High-fat food cravings can be caused by a deficiency of essential fatty acids. The body needs a constant supply of essential fatty acids to function properly. If you don't get enough, the body responds by ramping up cravings for any kind of fat. Getting enough essential fatty acids—which include alpha-linolenic acid (omega-3) and linoleic acid (omega-6) in foods that contain healthy fats—can reduce cravings for high-fat foods.

Don't Overdo It with Good Fats

Too much of a good thing can be counterproductive. Even though I recommend eating healthy fats, don't overdo it. Unhealthy fat and healthy fat have the same number of calories: 9 calories per gram. The difference is that unhealthy fats cause inflammation and leptin resistance. But when it comes to calorie counting, all fat is the same. So just because it has healthy fat doesn't mean you should eat a lot of it. I recommend that you keep your fat intake around 30 percent of daily calories (40 to 50 grams of fat daily for a 1,400-calorie diet).

Put the Brakes on Fast Food

It is best to avoid (or minimize) fast food. In addition to all that unhealthy fat, the typical fast food contains more than 1,000 calories and hundreds of milligrams of sodium. Researchers have found that even eating one fast food meal per week seriously impairs an individual's ability to maintain a healthy body weight over the long term.

STEP BY STEP

Make Better Meat Choices

If you are used to eating meat, it is unrealistic to completely stop eating it. You can reduce the amount of unhealthy fat you eat by following a few simple guidelines:

- Choose the healthiest cuts of meat.
  - -Beef: flank steak, top sirloin, bottom round steak, eye of round steak, sirloin tip side steak, and tenderloin
  - -Lamb: lean chops, roasts
  - -Pork: tenderloin, roasts
  - -Chicken and turkey: breast
- Don't eat meat with a marble-like texture or "prime" grade, which indicates a high amount of fat.
- Try healthier "free-range" or grass-fed instead of higher fat corn-fed beef.
- Trim all visible fat before cooking.
- Grill, broil, or bake and remove drippings.
- Have the butcher custom grind a healthy, lower fat cut of beef. Don't use prepackaged ground beef. Even "low-fat" preground ground beef is much higher in fat than if you have it ground yourself.
- Try low-fat "alternative" red meat, such as bison, elk, or ostrich.
- Try seafood instead of meat, or try "surf and turf" by cutting the meat portion in half and adding a broiled lobster tail or some steamed shrimp.
- Use ground chicken or turkey breast, instead of the regular variety, which contains some dark meat and skin.

Do You Have Essential Fatty Acid (EFA) Deficiency?

The essential fatty acids are necessary for health and wellness. EFA deficiency can lead to a variety of symptoms:

___ Cravings for high-fat foods
___ Painful or stiff joints
___ Dry, scaly, or flaky skin
___ Cracking or peeling fingertips
___ Small bumps on the back of upper arms
___ Thick or cracked calluses
___ Dandruff
___ Dry or brittle hair
___ Soft or splitting fingernails
___ Unexplained allergic reactions
___ Dry eyes
___ Dry mouth
___ Depression
___ Memory loss

If you have two or more of these symptoms, you could have EFA deficiency. Symptoms of EFA deficiency usually resolve a few weeks after adding more healthy fats to the diet.

Eat a Cup of Veggies before 10 a.m.

Try to make eating a cup of vegetables a morning ritual. Think of it as taking a vitamin or a supplement instead of being part of your diet. You can add vegetables to your breakfast, have them as a morning snack, or just wolf them down in a few bites. Most people who struggle with overeating don't eat enough vegetables. If you don't like eating vegetables, I have some advice: Eat them anyway; they won't kill you. Even if you don't do it every day, try it just one day.

WHAT DO YOU HAVE TO LOSE?

If you're asking why you should eat a cup of vegetables in the morning, I would ask you to consider any reasons for not doing it. What are the downsides, the

Beware of Nuts

The good: Nuts contain the healthiest fats.
The bad: Nuts are high in calories.
The ugly: Nuts can trigger binge eating.

Nuts contain healthy monounsaturated fats but are very high in calories and should be eaten in limited amounts. The best way to eat nuts is combined with other foods, as in crushed nuts on a salad or green beans with sliced almonds. Eating nuts all by themselves can trigger overeating because ounce for ounce they are extremely high in calories. If you snack on a small portion of nuts without any other foods, you may end up feeling even hungrier.

Vegetable Juices Don't Cut It

Drinking a can of vegetable juice is not as good as eating vegetables. Why? Juice contains liquid calories that aren't sensed by your gut hormones. Even though juice has a lot of vitamins and minerals, it has empty calories. Even homemade vegetable juice that contains a lot of fiber and pulp, while very healthy, has less of an impact on satisfying your gut hormones than eating the whole vegetables (see chapter 6). When it comes to your hunger hormones, you are better off eating vegetables instead of drinking juice. Commercial tomato juice and tomato vegetable juice blends are also very high in sodium, even the low-sodium varieties.

risks? The answer is: There is no downside. The only thing you have to lose is excess fat. Eating a full cup of vegetables in the morning and treating them as a nutritional supplement will help you beat overeating because they make you feel really full at the time of the day when your body needs fiber and volume.

Moreover, vegetables contain antioxidants that reduce inflammation, improve leptin resistance, and help you burn fat. The high vitamin and mineral content in vegetables also helps reduce cravings.

The idea of eating vegetables as a vitamin supplement was first recommended by Jackie Warner in her book *This Is Why You're Fat*. I have found this technique especially useful for my patients who hate eating vegetables. By viewing them as medication, it enables many of my patients to consume more vegetables than they would otherwise. I tell my patients this is just one more challenge for you to take on. It is one more "to-do" behavior to add to your repertoire. Even if you don't eat a full cup, eating any vegetables in the morning will be beneficial. Try eating just one cooked mushroom or a couple of baby carrots. Gradually increase the amount you eat over time.

STEP BY STEP

Ways to Get that Veggie Serving in

- Pre-portion fresh or frozen vegetables and keep them available at all times.
- Have microwave steamer bags or a microwave-safe container for cooking.
- Keep frozen, chopped broccoli (microwave for 90 seconds) in your freezer at home and at work.
- Mindlessly nibble on crunchy veggies, such as baby carrots, celery, green beans, or slices of bell pepper.
- Eat cooked, mashed yellow squash or zucchini seasoned with black pepper and garlic.
- Add fresh spinach to a fruit smoothie.
- Have a vegetable egg white omelet or frittata.
- Enjoy poached eggs with broiled mushrooms.
- Try a breakfast burrito with vegetables.
- Eat sliced tomatoes with a drop of olive oil on top.

Keep on Moving!

When I see patients with leptin resistance, I always emphasize regular exercise and physical activity as an important component of treatment. I recommend exercising every day, or as many days as possible. The more you exercise, the better the results.

In addition to formal exercise, increasing physical activity is also important. The definition of physical activity is moving your body through space. Any type of physical activity, like taking the stairs instead of the elevator, gardening, housekeeping, playing with the kids, or walking at the mall is beneficial. For people with sedentary jobs, I recommend walking around the office for a couple of minutes every hour during your work day.

CONSISTENT EXERCISE LEADS TO IDEAL WEIGHT

Consistent exercise, like a consistent diet, helps leptin stay balanced for the long term. Studies show that people who exercise regularly are most likely to be at their ideal body weight. Physical activity burns calories and boosts metabolism. It alleviates inflammation and is a powerful way to rapidly improve the way leptin functions in the body. Sitting too long at one time causes leptin resistance. The simple act of getting up for a minute or two every hour can help get leptin back on track (see chapter 9 for the best ways to make exercise and physical activity part of your daily routine).

Remember to Stay Hydrated

Our bodies are 70 percent water. Not drinking enough water causes leptin resistance and stops fat loss, even if you have a healthy diet. Good hydration helps burn fat by decreasing inflammation and helping your metabolic machinery function. Studies have shown that drinking a full glass of water before each meal lowers appetite.

I tell my patients to drink 2 quarts (1.9 L) of filtered water every day. Cold water helps boost metabolism because it forces the body to burn more calories to generate body heat, but it is okay to drink warm or hot beverages and other calorie-free beverages, such as flavored waters, sparkling water, unsweetened tea, or coffee.

Microwave Frozen Broccoli

Chopped broccoli is my favorite choice for a morning cup of vegetables. I can always find frozen chopped broccoli at my grocery store, and I just pop it in the microwave. A cup of broccoli has almost as much protein as an egg, and is high in fiber, low in calories, and superhigh in antioxidants. For a healthy thyroid, always cook your broccoli (see chapter 5).

1 cup of chopped broccoli contains:

- 30 calories
- 3 grams of protein
- 2 grams of fiber
- 150 mg of vitamin C

Look Out for Limes; They May Disrupt Hormones

Although it is perfectly fine to use lime as a flavoring from time to time, studies have shown that daily consumption of lime juice can disrupt hormones.

You should not drink sweetened beverages, such as sodas, juice, or sweet tea, because they are high in sugar and calories. Diet drinks and other artificially sweetened beverages should be consumed in limited amounts or avoided altogether. Numerous studies have linked artificial sweeteners to weight gain because the artificial sweetness combined with no calories confuses the brain into thinking that sugar is coming, but it never does. This results in hunger and sugar cravings that can last for hours or days.

Remembering to drink water can be difficult for some people. As we get older, we lose our sense of thirst. You can increase your fluid intake by keeping a water bottle with you. Invest in a good BPA-free water bottle, fill it in the morning, and take it with you as a matter of course. This way, you don't have to buy water and you have it nearby, encouraging you to drink freely throughout the day.

ADD THE MAGIC OF LEMON

I recommend adding lemon to your water. Drinking water with lemon helps your body refresh, detoxify, hydrate, and cool down at the same time. Adding lemon makes water easier to drink, helping to ensure you get all you need every day. Lemon in your water can also decrease the absorption of carbohydrates from the food you eat because of its high acid content. Citrus fruits, including lemon, contain vitamin C and other antioxidants, which can fight inflammation and curb appetite and cravings. Lemon purée adds fiber to the water, which helps reduce cravings and hunger.

STEP BY STEP

Ways to Add Lemon to Water

- Thoroughly wash lemons before using them.
- Add slices or wedges to a glass of ice water; drink small sips all day.
- Try drinking warm or hot water with a slice of lemon in a mug and sip like coffee.
- Drink green tea or black tea with lemon.
- Grind a whole lemon in a food processor to make lemon purée, which can be added to your water throughout the day.
- Freeze ice cubes with slices of lemon and add to a glass or water.

Get Enough Quality Sleep

Many people simply don't get enough sleep. You should be sleeping at least six to eight hours every night. A good night's sleep is critical for leptin to work properly. In fact, studies have shown that poor sleep causes both leptin deficiency and leptin resistance. Leptin has a circadian rhythm; it peaks at night when you sleep and is lower during the day. If your sleep is disrupted or you don't get enough sleep, the normal nighttime leptin surge is blunted, making you hungry and triggering overeating. Even a few nights of poor sleep can lower your leptin levels by as much as 25 percent.

If you have problems falling asleep or staying asleep, there is a lot you can do to improve the quality of your sleep. Good sleep is just like many healthy behaviors that don't always come naturally; it takes hard work (see chapter 10 for more on improving sleep).

Oysters: The Zinc Kings

Ounce for ounce, oysters have more zinc than any other food. You can get your daily allowance of zinc with just two or three oysters. Oysters are low in fat and high in protein, the ideal nutrient combination to fight leptin resistance.

Increase Your Intake of Zinc, Antioxidants, and Omega-3 Fatty Acids

Did you know that zinc enhances leptin production? Be aware of the amounts of zinc you consume, as well as antioxidants and omega-3 fatty acids that alleviate inflammation and leptin resistance.

TAKE ZINC TO BOOST LEPTIN PRODUCTION

Research has shown that people with zinc deficiency also have low leptin levels. Replacing zinc restores leptin production back to normal. Zinc does very little, however, in helping to alleviate the more serious problem for most people: leptin resistance.

You need to get 10 to 50 mg of zinc every day, either from the foods you eat or from a supplement. This is because zinc is necessary for leptin to be made properly. Zinc is an important mineral that is necessary for the proper functioning of cells, normal immune system function, brain function, and many other important body functions.

Most standard multivitamins contain about 10 mg of zinc. If you eat a lot of beans and whole grains, you need at least 20 mg of zinc every day because these foods contain substances called phytates that bind zinc and inhibit its absorption.

Soak Your Beans

You can increase the available zinc in dried beans by soaking them in water for several hours before cooking and allowing them to sit after soaking until sprouts form (see page 44).

Drinking a lot of alcohol can deplete the body of zinc. People with bowel problems, such as Crohn's disease, colitis, chronic diarrhea, or irritable bowel syndrome, typically need 20 to 50 mg of zinc because zinc may not be absorbed properly. Gastric bypass patients are at particular risk for zinc deficiency because it isn't absorbed well. Many of my patients who have had gastric bypass develop zinc deficiency among other vitamin and mineral deficiencies because their bowels don't absorb minerals correctly. If you have had gastric bypass surgery, you need to take a 25 to 50 mg zinc supplement daily.

Be careful not to take too much zinc. Excessive zinc consumption has been linked to increased appetite.

What is Your Zinc Level?

A simple blood test can be done to determine if you have too little, too much, or just the right amount of zinc in your body. Most doctors don't do this routinely, but will perform the test if you ask them to. An ideal zinc level is 75 to 150 µg/dL.

FOODS HIGH IN ZINC

- Beans
- Beef
- Cashews and almonds
- Chicken
- Dark chocolate
- Lamb
- Oysters
- Peanuts
- Sesame seeds and pumpkin seeds
- Wheat germ

CONSUME MORE ANTIOXIDANTS TO CALM INFLAMMATION

The more antioxidants you consume the better. One of the easiest ways to do this is to eat more vegetables and fruits. Whole fruits and vegetables contain hundreds, if not thousands, of antioxidants, many of which don't even have names. Eat a variety of different-colored vegetables and fruits, as discussed in chapter 3, and remember to eat a cup of vegetables in the morning as a nutritional supplement.

Coffee, black and green tea, red wine, and dark chocolate are also terrific sources of antioxidants. Coffee is high in antioxidants and has been linked to a decreased risk for a number of diseases, including diabetes and cancer. Black tea and green tea have been shown in countless studies to contain powerful antioxidant compounds. Tea antioxidants, called polyphenols, are much more potent than vitamin C or vitamin E in their ability to neutralize inflammation. Resveratrol and polyphenols, key antioxidants in red wine and the skins of red grapes, have also been reported to have a number of anti-inflammatory benefits.

Vitamin and mineral supplements, on the other hand, contain only the vitamins and minerals with antioxidant properties that are listed on the label. Whenever possible, I recommend using real food instead of supplements as the best way of increasing antioxidants.

A True Blue Food

Try to eat blueberries every day. Although fresh blueberries can be expensive or hard to find, frozen blueberries are inexpensive and readily available. Blueberries are a great source of antioxidants and flavanoids—compounds that have powerful anti-inflammatory properties. Putting frozen blueberries in a smoothie is a great way to get them into your diet. You can use them in recipes, thaw them and use as a topping on yogurt or fat-free cottage cheese, or try eating them frozen as a crunchy snack.

Recommended Daily Vitamins with Antioxidant Properties for Leptin Resistance

Vitamin C	500 to 1000 mg
Vitamin B_1 (Thiamine)	1.5 to 2 mg
Vitamin B_2 (Riboflavin)	3 to 8 mg
Vitamin B_3 (Niacin)	20 to 100 mg
Vitamin B_6	5 to 10 mg
Vitamin B_{12}	500 to 1000 mcg
Folic Acid	500 to 1000 mcg

SOOTHE INFLAMMATION WITH OMEGA-3 FATTY ACIDS

In addition to zinc and antioxidants, you should also eat more omega-3 fatty acids to alleviate inflammation and leptin resistance. You can get omega-3 fatty acids by eating fish or taking supplements. I recommend that you consume 1000 to 4000 mg of omega-3 fatty acids a day. Food and supplements contain a combination of eicosapentaenoic acid (EPA) and docosahexaenoic acid (DHA), which are the two main omega-3 fatty acids.

Resveratrol Preserves Health

Resveratrol is an antioxidant in red grape skins and red wine that has been reported to have numerous health benefits. While the jury is still out on the benefit of resveratrol supplements, increasing your intake of natural sources of resveratrol are your best bet. You can eat red or purple grapes or drink red wine. Blueberries, cranberries, and peanuts also contain small amounts of resveratrol.

A 4-ounce (115 g) serving of salmon, for example, contains 1500 to 2300 mg of omega-3 fatty acids. Wild salmon has more omega-3 fatty acids than farm-raised salmon. A good rule of thumb: The deeper the red color of the flesh, the more omega-3 fatty acids contained in the salmon. Flaxseed also contains omega-3 fatty acids but is not as helpful for reducing inflammation as fish oil.

Identify and Treat Infections in Your Body

As you know by now, having excess fat in your body is one of the most common causes of inflammation. Chronic infections and other medical conditions can cause inflammation and leptin resistance too. If you have an inflammatory medical disorder, it may be contributing to overeating.

There are many different symptoms of these disorders; the best way to find out if you have an inflammatory medical condition is to see your physician and get regular checkups. However, many infections aren't obvious to either the person that has the infection or even the doctor.

Take note of any symptoms you may be having. Check your temperature; a temperature of 99.8°F (37.7°C) to 100.8°F (38.2°C) is considered a low-grade fever, which could be an indicator of a hidden infection. Most infections are treated with antibiotics, antifungal medications, or antiviral medications; however, treatments can be complex and require an individualized approach. For difficult cases, an infectious disease specialist can be helpful.

Do You Have a Hidden Infection?

___ Abdominal pain or sensitive stomach
___ Burning during urination
___ Coughing
___ Diarrhea
___ Elevated white blood cell count
___ Eyes stuck shut in the morning
___ Foot pain, ingrown toenails, or foot ulcers
___ Foul-smelling gas

___ Frequent throat clearing
___ Headache
___ Joint pain
___ Low-grade fever
___ Muscle aches
___ Night sweats
___ Rash
___ Ringing in the ears
___ Shivering or chills
___ Sinus congestion or drainage
___ Sneezing
___ Sore throat
___ Swollen glands or lymph nodes
___ Tired all the time
___ Tooth or gum problems
___ Vaginal discharge

If you have any of these symptoms, you should see your physician to look for a hidden infection.

COMMON SOURCES OF INFECTIONS THAT CONTRIBUTE TO LEPTIN RESISTANCE

- Chronic acne
- Chronic appendicitis
- Chronic bronchitis
- Chronic hepatitis
- Cuts and wounds
- Food poisoning
- Foot infections, ingrown toenails
- Frequent colds and flu
- Gallbladder problems
- Gingivitis
- Intestinal parasites, bacterial overgrowth
- Lyme disease
- Pelvic inflammatory disease
- Recurrent herpes, cold sores
- Sinus infections
- Tooth abscess
- Urinary tract infections
- Vaginal yeast infections

The Power of an Apple

Eating an apple a day is a good way to keep the doctor away—and lose weight. Many studies have shown the antioxidant properties and health benefits of apples, which are high in fiber, vitamin C, and flavanoids. Plus, one medium apple is only 80 calories!

Relief for the Burps

Some people complain of fishy-tasting belching from taking fish oil capsules. Many of my patients have found that freezing the capsules helps reduce this side effect. Another option is to ask your doctor to prescribe Lovaza, a prescription formulation of omega-3 fatty acids that is more purified and may result in fewer fishy burps.

CHRONIC CONDITIONS CAN CAUSE LEPTIN RESISTANCE

Chronic infections, also known as occult infections, are a common but frequently unrecognized cause of inflammation. The substances produced by our immune systems to fight infection have a nasty side effect of causing leptin resistance. When infections are treated, leptin resistance improves, allowing you to burn fat and feel more energetic.

CHRONIC INFLAMMATORY CONDITIONS THAT CONTRIBUTE TO LEPTIN RESISTANCE

- Arthritis
- Asthma
- Chronic kidney disease
- Diabetes, prediabetes, and insulin resistance
- Fatty liver disease
- Heart disease
- High blood pressure
- Inflammatory bowel disease
- Lupus
- Obesity, excess body fat
- Polycystic ovary syndrome
- Psoriasis

The Link between Leptin and Cancer

There is a growing body of scientific research linking obesity to cancer. Scientists are trying to understand what causes this link. In the lab, leptin has been shown to promote growth of cancer cells. The heavier a person is, the more leptin they make. Leptin has also been shown to promote breast cancer growth in mice. Experts believe that leptin is just one of many hormonal connections between obesity and cancer.

Get Back on Track as Soon as Possible

Beating overeating for long-term weight loss requires focus and commitment. When you deviate from your plan, it is important not to get too far off track. Just because you fell off the wagon doesn't mean you need to stay off. No one is perfect, and you have to be forgiving of yourself. Your hormones know this, and can deal with minor diversions. But if you get off track, you must pay attention so that you can get yourself back on track as soon as possible. When you get back on track quickly, you will be less likely to regain the weight you have lost.

STICK TO THE BON! EATING PLAN

The key to an optimal set point is having a stable, balanced diet. Unhealthy foods are not much of a problem if you only eat them on rare occasions. When eating unhealthy foods becomes a habit, your weight and set point creep up, coinciding with leptin resistance. Yo-yo dieting worsens the problem, making it more and more difficult to lose weight on subsequent attempts. Each time you lose weight and regain, your set point becomes more fixed at a higher body weight. The body strives to maintain this higher weight. By focusing on the long term, you can eventually reset your set point back to normal.

Be Your Own Patient Advocate

Chronic medical problems can be difficult to diagnose. The more you know about your own symptoms, the better you can communicate with your physician. Keep a record of symptoms you are having and bring the list to your doctor appointment. You should research your symptoms and the conditions I've mentioned here on the Internet, but be sure to use reliable medical websites (see chapter 10 for recommended websites).

CHAPTER 8

Avoid Endocrine System Disruptors

We live in a world filled with chemicals. Our drinking water is polluted with trace amounts of chemicals and pharmaceuticals. Our food supply is tainted by pesticides, hormones, preservatives, and additives. Food is stored in plastic containers and cooked in nonstick cookware that leach out contaminants. We breathe in secondhand smoke, car exhaust, and fumes from carpets and cleaning products. There are chemicals in cosmetics, antibacterial soap, and the flame-retardant fabrics used in our children's car seats and pajamas.

There is a growing body of research about how these chemicals are making people fat. The information is so new that word hasn't gotten out yet.

Until recently, experts have believed that excess food consumption and lack of exercise were the root causes of our current obesity epidemic. However, new research has also implicated endocrine-disrupting chemicals known as "environmental obesogens" that cause people to gain weight by increasing their appetite, lowering their metabolism, and stimulating their fat cells to multiply and grow larger.

*action*plan

Avoid Endocrine Disruptors

- *Drink clean water.*
- *Eat clean vegetables and fruits.*
- *Eat hormone-free meat and low-fat dairy products.*
- *Eat less fatty meat.*
- *Eat uncontaminated seafood.*
- *Flush out toxins.*
- *Cook and store food safely to minimize BPA and phthalate exposure.*
- *Wash your hands at least four times daily.*
- *Reduce skin contact with chemicals.*
- *Limit foods that contain natural endocrine disruptors.*

No one thinks these chemicals alone are responsible for the obesity epidemic. Experts believe that obesogens make people more susceptible to the effects of lack of exercise and a high-calorie diet. Modern society, which combines these chemicals with high-calorie food and all the conveniences that keep us sedentary, is like a perfect storm that leads to obesity.

THE DISCOVERY OF OBESOGENS

The endocrine system is a group of glands and organs that produce, store, and secrete hormones that control the growth, development, and metabolism of the body. Over the past twenty years, our understanding of how endocrine disruptors interfere with hormonal balance has grown substantially. The U.S. Environmental Protection Agency (EPA) has defined an endocrine-disrupting chemical as "an exogenous agent that interferes with . . . natural blood-borne hormones that are present in the body."

Are You Being Exposed to Endocrine Disruptors?

___ Do you drink unfiltered tap water?
___ Do you drink less than 2 quarts (1.9 L) of water daily?
___ Is your diet low in fresh fruits and vegetables?
___ Do you use plastic food containers or plastic wrap?
___ Do you eat a lot of canned goods?
___ Do you eat meat and dairy products that contain hormones?
___ Do you eat a lot of fatty meats?
___ Do you consume less than 25 to 35 grams of fiber daily?
___ Do you eat a lot of processed foods or restaurant foods?
___ Do you wash your hands infrequently?
___ Does your skin come in contact with chemicals?
___ Do you consume a lot of soy products?
___ Do you eat a lot of raw cruciferous vegetables?

If you answered yes to any of these questions, you can benefit from the action plan in this chapter.

Understand the Chemical Anarchy Within

Research has shown that on a cellular level, chemicals act in many different ways, all conspiring to disturb our delicate endocrine systems. Although some endocrine disruptors are substances that occur naturally in our environment (for example, cruciferous vegetables that block thyroid function, which I discuss in chapter 5), many others are synthetic chemicals.

This group of substances is highly diverse and includes chemicals used in plastic and plasticizers, such as bisphenol A (BPA) and phthalates, lubricants, and solvents, such as polychlorinated biphenyls (PCBs) and polybrominated biphenyls (PBBs), and pesticides and fungicides (the "cides"). These compounds disrupt sex hormones and are toxic to the thyroid gland. Mercury and other heavy metals have also been found to disrupt thyroid and sex hormone balance, on top of all the other bad things these compounds are known to do.

In today's world, it is impossible to completely avoid chemicals. Take lead for example. Lead paint and leaded gasoline have been banned for decades because of their known toxic effects, but even today, 1.4 percent of children have unacceptably high levels of lead in their blood. PCBs were banned in the 1970s but are still found in the blood of Americans today, even in children who were born after the ban took effect. These chemicals, still in our environment, find ways of creeping into our bodies.

Endocrine-disrupting chemicals from pollutants and pesticides seep deep into the soil and end up in the water supply. Perchlorate (a pollutant) and atrazine (a pesticide) are thyroid toxins that have been found in drinking water. Arsenic, lead, and many other toxins can contaminate drinking water as well.

THE BUZZ ABOUT BISPHENOL A (BPA) AND PHTHALATES

BPA is an endocrine-disrupting chemical found in plastics that has been linked to weight gain, which I'll discuss later in this chapter. Ninety-three percent of Americans have detectable levels of BPA in their urine. BPA is also found in dust, dental fillings, toys, and thermal cash register receipts. BPA is best known for its ability to imitate and disrupt the hormone estrogen; however, it also has an effect on stimulating fat cell growth. In addition to weight gain, studies have linked BPA to infertility, early puberty, prostate cancer, breast cancer, and diabetes. There is belief that BPA may rewire the body's fat cell production system, making it produce increased numbers of larger fat cells.

Drink Lemon Water to Rid Yourself of Toxins

Toxins persist and concentrate in tissues in the body, building up over time. Most toxins accumulate in fat and stay there for a long time. When you lose weight, these toxins can be released, making you feel lousy and your body resist losing weight. I recommend drinking 2 quarts (1.9 L) of filtered water, flavored with real lemon (a natural diuretic), to keep your metabolism humming while you flush the toxins out.

Phthalates are another hormone-disrupting chemical found in plastics. Researchers from Switzerland have called phthalates "metabolic disruptors" because they stimulate receptors that make fat cells grow and list them as a possible contributor to the obesity epidemic.

Many new products are labeled BPA- and phthalate-free. The concern is that the replacement plastics are untested and may pose equal or even more harm. We just don't know. Minimizing exposure to all plastics is your best bet.

A PRIME OFFENDER IN PVC

Tributyltin is a potent obesogen found in PVC pipe. It is also found in fungicides. Tributyltin stimulates production of new and larger fat cells, boosts appetite, raises cortisol levels, and inhibits estrogen. We don't really know how much tributyltin gets into the water from PVC pipe, but even a miniscule amount can pose a risk. Previously, no one realized that tributyltin did any harm at all. Now, there is a huge amount of scientific data suggesting that tributyltin is one of the most potent obesogens that we know of.

One of the ways that tributyltin makes you fat is by stimulating a cellular receptor known as peroxisome proliferator-activated receptor-gamma, or PPAR-gamma (pronounced *pee-par gamma*) for short. The PPAR-gamma receptor is also the target for the diabetes medications pioglitazone and rosiglitazone, which are known obesogens (see chapter 10 for more on obesogenic medicines). Many of my patients who have taken PPAR-gamma medications have gained a huge amount of weight as a side effect. Because of this (and other side effects), use of this class of medications has been on the decline.

Reduce Your Exposure to Chemicals

It may not be realistic to avoid chemicals entirely, but there is a lot you can do to reduce your exposure.

Drink Clean Water

Not all drinking water is contaminated, but tap water can potentially contain hundreds of contaminants, some of which can make you fat. Even filtered water can become contaminated from the container it is kept in. I recommend using filtered water whenever possible, and keep it in a glass or stainless steel container. You need to drink at least 2 quarts (1.9 L) of clean, pure water every day.

A whole-house water purifier will eliminate 99 percent of contaminants from all of the water in your home, but this a very expensive solution. I also like the water purifiers that can be installed into a faucet, or a dispenser next to the faucet, or in the refrigerator.

Take care to clean water purifiers and replace filters according to the manufacturer's instructions. Most plastic water filter/pitcher products like Brita and PUR are BPA-free; however, they are still made of plastic. It's better to use these to filter the water, then transfer it to a glass container for storage. Even some aluminum water bottles contain BPA. Most bottled water is low in contaminants and a good choice when stored in glass or BPA-free plastic.

Drink a Lot of Water When Losing Weight

Throughout this book, I have discussed the importance of keeping yourself hydrated by drinking 2 quarts (1.9 L) of water daily, which is especially important when you are losing weight. Water loss is a natural consequence of losing weight, and if you don't increase the water you are drinking, the result will be dehydration, and your metabolic machinery won't be able to function at peak performance. Water also helps keep your appetite low, as I discuss in chapter 3.

Eat Clean Vegetables and Fruits

Eating clean vegetables and fruits requires washing them, but you should do more than just rinse them off. Vegetables and fruits are the healthiest foods you can eat, but they can contain chemicals that disrupt your hormones and cause you to gain weight. The main contaminants of fruits and vegetables are pesticides known as organophosphates, as well as BPA and phthalates from plastic packaging. Here are some suggestions to reduce the amount of hormone-disrupting chemicals in your vegetables and fruits.

SOAK AND RINSE VEGETABLES AND FRUITS

Washing vegetable and fruits helps remove pesticides and herbicides as well as BPA and other chemicals from the packaging. Wash all packaged vegetables and fruits even if the label says prewashed and ready to eat. Sprays and other vegetable cleaning products are available, but there is no proof that they are any better than plain water.

Soak fruits and vegetables in a large bowl of water for a minute or two. Use a lot of water and completely submerge the vegetables and fruits, then rinse them under running water. Use a colander for berries, small fruits, and vegetables. You can use a soft brush to lightly scrub hard surfaces such as citrus,

Grow Your Own Vegetables

Growing your own organic vegetables is a great way to ensure you are getting produce that is free of pesticides. Make sure to wash homegrown vegetables thoroughly.

apples, melons, peppers, and cucumbers. Wash all the parts of the vegetable or fruit, even if it is a part you don't plan to eat. Remove bruised or damaged areas of vegetables and fruits.

KEEP COUNTERTOPS, CUTLERY, AND COOKWARE CLEAN

BPA and other toxins can accumulate in dust and settle on countertops, cutlery, and cookware. Rinse off cookware with running water before using it. Wipe off countertops frequently. Clean a knife with a damp cloth before using it.

EAT FRESH FOODS

BPA and phthalates in plastic food containers and the linings of cans can contaminate food and beverages. Eating fresh or frozen foods as often as possible will reduce your exposure. One study showed that eating fresh foods can reduce BPA levels by more than 50 percent within a few days. Fresh vegetables (not wrapped in plastic wrap) have the lowest levels of BPA. Canned and frozen vegetables tend to have higher BPA levels because of the packaging.

DON'T BUY FRESH FRUITS AND VEGETABLES PACKED IN PLASTIC WRAP

Ironically, fresh fruits and vegetables packaged with plastic wrap can have high BPA levels from the plastic wrap.

LOOK FOR BPA-FREE CANS

Some companies are using BPA-free linings for their cans. Hain, Eden Foods, Celestial, ConAgra, and H.J. Heinz have all changed to BPA-free linings for some products. Be sure to read the labels.

BUY ORGANIC VEGETABLES AND FRUITS WHEN POSSIBLE

Thin-skinned vegetables and fruits can absorb a lot of toxins, as can green, leafy vegetables. Washing does not remove all the toxins. In fact, even peeled vegetables and fruits have been found to contain toxins. The vegetables and fruits listed below are the worst offenders when it comes to toxins. I recommend buying organic versions of these vegetables and fruits whenever possible.

THE DIRTY DOZEN

- Apples
- Celery
- Strawberries
- Peaches
- Spinach
- Nectarines
- Grapes (imported)
- Sweet bell peppers
- Potatoes
- Blueberries
- Lettuce
- Kale/collard greens

Source: Environmental Working Group

VEGETABLES AND FRUITS LOWEST IN PESTICIDES

- Onions
- Sweet corn
- Pineapples
- Avocados
- Asparagus
- Sweet peas
- Mangoes
- Eggplant
- Cantaloupe
- Kiwi
- Cabbage
- Watermelon
- Sweet potatoes
- Grapefruit
- Mushrooms

Source: Environmental Working Group

MSG Causes Weight Gain

Monosodium glutamate (MSG) is a flavor enhancer that has been linked to weight gain. In a study published in the *American Journal of Clinical Nutrition*, researchers from the University of North Carolina at Chapel Hill found that MSG caused weight gain in subjects they studied. We don't know exactly why MSG causes weight gain, but scientists speculate that MSG may cause leptin resistance (see chapter 7) by damaging appetite centers in the brain.

Buy Homemade Canned Goods

Before we had so many canned goods, people had to do their own canning, storing cooked vegetables in jars. Research your area for farmers' markets or specialty food stores where homemade canned goods in glass jars are sold. Or consider taking up a new hobby: canning your own vegetables.

Use Dried Beans Instead of Canned Beans

Even canned organic beans can contain BPA. Make your own homemade beans from dried beans using the recipe in chapter 2.

Eat Hormone-Free Meat and Dairy Products

Farmers use a lot of hormones in their livestock, especially cattle, to produce larger animals or to help them produce more milk. These hormones (administered to the animals by injection) are considered species-specific, meaning that cow hormones aren't supposed to work in humans.

Most of the animal hormones get digested when you consume them and are generally thought to pose little risk to humans. However, no one really knows if these hormones are having any effect in the people who consume them. I recommend minimizing exposure to animal hormones whenever possible.

Buy lean, hormone-free meat and dairy products. Meats and dairy products that are labeled organic do not contain hormones. You can also find meats and dairy products that are hormone free but may not be organic.

You don't have to devote your life to eating only organic foods, but whenever you do have a choice, try to choose organic or hormone-free meats and dairy products.

Eat Less Fatty Meat

Even if the meat is organic or hormone-free, you should limit your consumption of fatty red meat. As I discuss in chapter 7, there are a lot of ways you can decrease the fatty content in the meat you eat, including choosing leaner cuts of meat and trying alternative low-fat red meat, such as bison, venison, or elk.

Fatty meat, especially red meat, can contain high amounts of PCBs, or polychlorinated biphenyls, which tend to concentrate in the fat of grazing animals. PCBs are pollutants that were banned in the 1970s and are still in our environment. PCBs cause weight gain and a number of other hormone disruptions. Among the toxic effects, PCBs are an obesogen that cause fat cells to grow and multiply. Studies have found that people with higher levels of PCBs are more likely to develop type 2 diabetes. It is thought that PCBs induce insulin resistance and stimulate the pancreas to secrete higher amounts of insulin, which can stimulate hunger centers in the brain. PCBs also have been found to cause inflammation, which leads to leptin resistance (see chapter 7), and lead to increased risk of cardiovascular disease.

Eat Uncontaminated Seafood

You don't need to stop eating fish, but you should make an effort to eat more seafood with less mercury content and eat less fish with high mercury content, such as mackerel, shark, and swordfish. A good rule of thumb is the larger the fish, the higher the mercury content.

Fish are generally considered a healthy food—high in protein, vitamin B_{12}, and omega-3 fatty acids. But eating fish contaminated with mercury can be hazardous to your health, and may even cause you to gain weight. There has been a lot of concern about mercury in fish.

The mercury in fish is in the form of methylmercury, a potent neurotoxin formed by plankton, which is consumed and concentrated up the food chain. We have known of the bad things mercury can do, such as causing neurological damage, for a long time. But new research suggests that on top of all the known toxicities, mercury may also be an endocrine disruptor interfering with thyroid hormone and sex hormone receptors. There is not a lot of research on mercury consumption and body weight, but given its known toxicities, I advise that you limit your exposure.

MERCURY LEVELS IN SEAFOOD

High Mercury

- Mackerel (King)
- Shark
- Swordfish
- Tilefish

Intermediate Mercury

- Chilean bass
- Grouper
- Halibut
- Lobster
- Mackerel (Spanish)
- Orange roughy
- Tuna

(continued on next page)

Low Mercury

- Anchovies
- Catfish
- Clams
- Cod
- Crab
- Crawfish
- Haddock
- Herring
- Oysters
- Perch
- Pollock
- Salmon
- Scallops
- Squid
- Tilapia
- Trout

Adapted from www.fda.gov

Flush Out the Toxins

Drinking plenty of water and eating foods that are high in fiber is the best way to dilute and eliminate toxins in your body.

To flush out toxins, eat foods high in fiber, such as vegetables, fruits, whole grains, and high-fiber cereals. You should consume 25 to 35 grams of fiber every day. If you can't get enough fiber in your diet, take a supplement. Exercising regularly and drinking at least 2 quarts (1.9 L) of water daily also help.

Fiber, a Trusted Transport

Eating more fiber allows your bowels to function better. Studies have shown that eating more fresh fruits and vegetables and other plant-based foods helps flush the body of PCBs and other toxins. Fiber results in a well-formed, soft, and easily passed stool. Rapid transit and elimination of stool out of the body means that the chemicals in your food are passed more quickly through the system. Toxins don't have as much opportunity to get absorbed through the bowel wall. Fewer endocrine-disrupting chemicals and other harmful substances have time to get absorbed. This is also why a high-fiber diet reduces the risk for colon cancer. See chapter 6 for more information on a high-fiber diet.

Cook and Store Food Safely to Minimize Exposure

Following a few simple tips can reduce the amount of BPA and phthalates you are exposed to when you cook and store food.

USE GLASS OR STAINLESS STEEL CONTAINERS

This is especially important for storing high-fat foods and acidic foods that tend to collect more chemicals from plastic containers than other foods.

NEVER MICROWAVE FOOD IN PLASTIC

Even "microwave safe" plastic containers leach out BPA. Heating plastic containers puts even more chemicals into your food.

AVOID PLASTIC WRAP

Try not to buy fruits and vegetables that are packaged in plastic wrap. Remove all wrapping as soon as possible.

MAKE COFFEE THE OLD-FASHIONED WAY

Use a French press or old-fashioned percolator to make coffee. Most automatic coffee makers contain BPA and phthalates in their tubing.

Wash Your Hands at Least Four Times Daily

Several times a day, wash your hands under lukewarm running water for at least twenty seconds using regular soap. Do not substitute using hand sanitizer or antibacterial wipes for soap and water when washing your hands.

A study done at Boston University School of Public Health measured levels of polybrominated diphenyl ethers (PBDEs) in offices throughout the Boston area. PBDEs are hormone-disrupting chemicals used as flame retardants. Workers who washed their hands four or more times daily had lower levels of *PBDEs* in their blood.

Most manufacturers stopped using PBDEs in their products in 2004, but the chemicals they use in its place are untested and may have the same effect. In addition, PBDEs remain in the older products we still use every day, such as office chairs, carpeting, and computers. PBDEs get stored in fat tissue and can stay there for years. PBDEs can be found everywhere; they are in dust and all over our homes and offices.

Cloves Cleanse Toxins from Your Body

A chemical compound in cloves known as eugenol is thought to help flush toxins and cleanse the body of environmental pollutants. Cloves are high in manganese and vitamin C, and contain omega-3 fatty acids. They also have antioxidant and anti-inflammatory properties.

PBDEs are just an example; there are many chemicals that are removed when you wash your hands. You can't avoid chemicals completely, but washing your hands helps lower the amount of chemicals that get absorbed into your body through the skin on your hands.

REDUCE SKIN CONTACT WITH CHEMICALS

Chemicals in the environment can get absorbed through your skin. Here are a few tips for reducing the amount of endocrine-disrupting chemicals that get absorbed through your skin.

THROW AWAY YOUR THERMAL CASH REGISTER RECEIPTS

Most people know about reducing BPA exposure by avoiding plastic containers and wraps, but did you know that the thermal register tape used by most retailers and restaurants contain BPA? Thermal cash register receipts contain a lot of BPA, although efforts are being made to develop BPA-free thermal paper. Once you've made note of a transaction in your records, tear up your receipt, throw it away, and wash your hands afterward.

WATCH OUT FOR FLAME RETARDANTS

PBDE (as discussed above) is a flame retardant and an endocrine system disruptor that manufacturers stopped using in 2004, but remains in our homes and offices today. Other flame retardants are also of concern.

Three decades ago, a flame retardant called brominated Tris was banned from children's pajamas because of health risks. Today, a similar flame retardant is still being used in baby products, such as car seats, high chairs, and nursing pillows. The chemical, chlorinated Tris, has been thought to cause thyroid dysfunction. The Consumer Product Safety Commission now says that Tris flame retardants "may pose a significant risk to health consumers."

No one really knows how much chlorinated Tris is absorbed into the body. Manufacturers argue that the chemical is worth the risk because it makes products safer if they catch fire. Unfortunately, there is no requirement for manufacturers to label products that contain fire retardants or to list the chemicals they use.

DON'T USE ANTIBACTERIAL SOAP

Antibacterial soap contains the chemical triclosan, which acts as an endocrine disruptor by decreasing production of thyroid hormone, estrogen, and testosterone. Regular soap is equally effective in reducing germs on your hands without the hormone-disrupting effect.

AVOID CONTACT WITH WEED KILLERS

The compound glyphosate, found in chemical weed killers, can act as a thyroid hormone disruptor.

Limit Foods that Contain Natural Endocrine Disruptors

Two categories of foods contain natural hormone-disrupting substances: cruciferous vegetables and soy products.

Cruciferous vegetables, known as goitrogens (see chapter 5), contain a thyroid toxin, and when consumed uncooked in large amounts, can disrupt thyroid hormone function. Limit consumption of raw vegetables, including cabbage, broccoli, brussels sprouts, turnips, rutabaga, mustard, kohlrabi, radishes, cauliflower, cassava, millet, and kale to three or four servings per week. These vegetables pose no harm when cooked, so eat unlimited amounts of cooked.

The second category is the estrogen-like substances that are found naturally in plants. Known as phytoestrogens or isoflavones, these plant estrogens include genistein and coumestrol. More than three hundred different foods contain phytoestrogens, but the main foods are soy and products made from soy, such as tofu, soy milk, and soy baby formula. Limit soy products to two or three servings per week for men and children, five or six servings per week for women, and six or seven servings per week for women in menopause. Unless babies have severe allergy or intolerance to milk, soy-based baby formulas should be avoided altogether.

Other foods that contain tiny amounts of phytoestrogens include lentils, whole-grain wheat, rice, dates, flaxseed, bean sprouts, pomegranates, cherries, coffee, garlic, and thyme. These foods don't have enough phytoestrogens to do any harm.

Choose Whey Protein Over Soy Protein

For weight loss, whey or milk protein is better than soy protein, according to researchers from the U.S. Department of Agriculture's Human Nutrition Research Center. In a study of overweight and obese adults, researchers compared protein shakes made from soy protein and whey protein. The shakes had the same number of calories and percentages of carbohydrate and protein. The only difference was the type of protein: soy or whey.

After six months, participants who drank the soy shakes hadn't lost any weight compared to those who drank a nutritionally similar whey protein shake who lost a couple of pounds. The group who drank the soy drink had no change in their waistline,

(cont. right)

Soy and the Thyroid

Besides disrupting sex hormones, soy can disrupt the thyroid. Soy has been shown to interfere with an enzyme known as thyroid peroxidase, which is responsible for an important step in the production of thyroid hormone. The National Center for Toxicological Research reports that soy isoflavones have a number of antithyroid effects resulting in "soy toxicity."

A study from England found that soy phystoestrogen supplementation increased the risk for an underactive thyroid threefold. Another study from the University of Belgrade showed that soy isoflavones cause changes in the thyroid tissue leading to decreased thyroid hormone production.

THE ROLE OF ESTROGEN IN WEIGHT GAIN

Research has shown that the estrogen-like compounds in soy products can stimulate fat cells to grow and multiply. We know that estrogen can stimulate the body to make more fat tissue. For example, high-dose birth control pills that contain high amounts of estrogen have weight gain as a known side effect. Other research has shown that the effect can depend on the amount consumed and whether you are a man or a woman.

In men, natural estrogens tend to cause weight gain. In women, consumption of soy foods can cause weight gain, but higher doses of soy phytoestrogens found in soy menopause supplements may cause fat loss. A study from Italy found that high doses of the soy compound genistein can decrease fat tissue in female mice when used at doses equivalent to a menopausal supplement, but when used at the dose similar to eating soy foods, the mice gained fat.

Soy baby formula may especially be worrisome because of new research showing a greater impact on babies. Previously, it was thought that soy-based formula posed no harm to infants, but this wisdom is being reconsidered. Infants who are fed soy formula have concentrations of phytoestrogens in their body that are five hundred times higher than those fed cow's milk formula. Scientists don't even know what this means or what this does to these babies because very little research has been done.

Soy products also have health benefits, especially for women, so they don't need to be avoided altogether. Phytoestrogen consumption has been shown to have beneficial effects in women with diabetes by improving the way insulin works. They have also been shown to reduce risk factors for cardiovascular disease, especially in women after menopause. We still have a lot to learn about natural estrogens and how they affect body weight and fat cells.

but those who drank whey lost about an inch (2.5 cm) around the middle. The researchers speculated that the difference in weight loss between the two groups may have to do with lower ghrelin levels and feeling more satisfied, which were seen in the subjects who drank whey protein shakes compared to those drinking a soy shake. Other endocrine effects of soy protein—such as changes in estrogen and thyroid hormone—may also play a role in the lack of weight loss experienced by the subjects who drank soy shakes.

Questions that Need Answers

Scientists are just beginning to understand the health repercussions of exposure to the unnatural substances that bombard our bodies on a daily basis. It is difficult to do research in this area because we are exposed to so many chemicals that it is tough to determine what chemicals are doing what damage. The Centers for Disease Control and Prevention (CDC) has been monitoring blood and urine samples from about 2,500 people who live in different parts of the country to help understand what substances we are exposed to. We know that there are measurable amounts of at least three hundred chemicals in our bodies.

There is a big difference in knowing what chemicals we are exposed to and what harm they are doing. Until recently, there was debate that these chemicals were even getting into our bodies. This debate is over. Many questions remain:

- What are they doing to our bodies and to our hormones?
- What are the medical and health consequences of long-term exposure?
- How do these chemicals make us hungrier and make our fat cells grow out of control?

The CDC has said that we really don't know the extent of the health risk from all these chemicals. Human experiments to answer this question are not ethical and will never be done. Some studies can be done looking retrospectively, but a lot of what we know now and will know in the future about these substances comes from animal studies and basic laboratory research.

The reality is that we are all part of a grand experiment. These chemicals are in our food supply and in our environment. They are in your body, circulating in your bloodstream and permeating your tissues. We are all waiting to find out the long-term effects of these substances.

PART THREE:
Bring on the Reinforcements

CHAPTER

9

Beat Overeating with Exercise

Overeating high-calorie foods is not the only reason people gain weight. Decreased calorie burning from having a sedentary lifestyle or a sedentary occupation is the major contributor to the obesity epidemic over the past fifty years, according to research done by Dr. Timothy Church and his colleagues at Louisiana State University.

Ten thousand years ago, humans walked or ran 12 to 14 miles (19 to 22.5 km) each day. Our bodies are designed to move all the time, every day. Our lifestyle and work have become less physically demanding over the past five decades. Jobs have shifted from manufacturing and agriculture to high-tech and service.

The average number of calories burned in a day has decreased by 120 to 140 calories per day. This change alone may account for a large portion of the obesity epidemic we are experiencing. Even though it may seem like a small change, researchers estimate this translates to a 30-pound (14 kg) weight gain for the average individual.

Changing your occupation to a more physically demanding one may not be realistic, but adding some moderate or vigorous physical activity to your day can compensate for this decrease in calories burned.

***action*plan**

Exercise Daily

- *Be aware of your long-term goal.*
- *Do fat-burning exercises.*
- *Do muscle-building exercises.*
- *Exercise in the morning.*
- *Try multiple bouts of exercise in a day.*
- *Have fun.*
- *Strengthen neck and chest muscles.*
- *Exercise in the water.*
- *Eat a light slow-carb snack before you exercise.*
- *Push yourself.*

Build Your Stamina and Muscles

As with eating healthy foods, when it comes to exercise, it's important to mix it up. Be sure to get in a combination of aerobic fat-burning exercise and anaerobic muscle-building exercise. According to the CDC, only 12 percent of people get enough of both of these types of exercise.

Exercise is important for losing weight, but even more important when it comes to weight maintenance. According to the National Weight Control Registry, 94 percent of people who have lost weight and kept it off did so by increasing exercise. Ninety percent of these people exercise sixty minutes or more every day. Consistent daily aerobic exercise boosts metabolism and alleviates insulin and leptin resistance.

Besides helping you lose weight and keep it off, regular exercise can help you feel better and be healthier. Studies have shown that exercising reduces the risk for health problems, including cardiovascular disease (heart attacks and strokes), diabetes, sleep apnea, high blood pressure, bone loss, and even cancer. Regular exercise reduces the frequency and severity of the common cold by more than 40 percent.

TURN BACK THE CLOCK

Consistent daily exercise also slows aging and helps you live longer. Not exercising every day, on the other hand, makes you vulnerable to overeating by slowing metabolism and increasing leptin resistance and insulin resistance.

In one study by researchers at McMaster University in Ontario, mice who exercised regularly showed remarkable anti-aging effects, including darker, thicker fur, more muscle mass, and larger brain volume. The mice also showed significant improvements in the functioning of their mitochondria, a part of the cell that naturally degenerates with aging. The more physically fit you are, the greater the anti-aging benefit.

Exercise not only strengthens the body, it strengthens the mind. Countless studies have shown the benefits on the brain: better memory, energy level, and test scores. Exercise decreases anxiety and depression, and it is one of the best forms of stress reduction. Exercise raises levels of an important brain chemical known as brain-derived neurotrophic factor (BDNF). This substance makes brain cells grow and thrive. Dr. John Ratey, author of *Spark: The Revo-*

lutionary New Science of Exercise and the Brain, calls BDNF "Miracle-Gro" for the brain because of these effects.

Be Aware of Your Long-Term Goal

If you are just beginning an exercise program, start slowly with a challenging, but realistic goal. Even moderate-intensity physical activity of just five to ten minutes per day can add up and make a big difference. The key is not to overdo it. Gradually build up the time and intensity of your exercise with a goal of exercising every single day.

Your long-term goal is to exercise sixty to ninety minutes every day. Any exercise is beneficial, and doing more of it is even better. One of my patients has made all-day hikes his regular routine at least once each weekend. He hikes six to eight hours in a typical day, burning over a thousand calories each time.

As you build new healthy habits into your daily routine, you can add exercise to work up to this goal. Even if you start out exercising for one or two minutes a day, you can build up slowly to the long-term goal. It is important to have a goal of exercising every day. It is okay to take a day off from time to time, but don't deviate too far from this goal.

If you are already doing very intense workouts, such as jogging, biking, or swimming, where your heart rate is between 140 and 170 beats per minute (to the point where you are breathing heavily), you can shorten the daily goal to forty-five to sixty minutes. According to the CDC, one minute of vigorous physical activity equals two minutes of moderate-intensity physical activity. Regardless of the level of intensity, exercising longer is even better.

MIDDLE-AGED OR AT RISK? SEE YOUR DOCTOR FIRST

Exercise is the best thing most people can do for their heart. However, before getting started, doctors recommend that people over the age of thirty-five—or those who are overweight or have other risk factors for heart disease, such as high blood pressure, high cholesterol, diabetes, or a family history of heart disease—receive exercise clearance from a physician before beginning an exercise program.

STEP BY STEP

Ways to Plan for Daily Exercise

- Keep a journal or chart for exercise.
- Write down specific times you will exercise.
- Write down what exercise you will do.
- Write down what you need to do this (i.e., get dressed, drive to gym, etc.).
- Problem-solve any potential issues that could stop you from doing the next day's exercise.
- Write down alternate exercises as a backup (i.e., raining, gym closed, class canceled, etc.).
- Mark off completed exercise in your journal or chart and review often.

In addition to asking about any symptoms and performing a physical examination, and checking your pulse and blood pressure, your doctor may do additional testing. Most people get an electrocardiogram (EKG), which is a paper tracing of the electrical impulses of the heart. Some doctors will recommend a treadmill stress test, which is where you walk on a treadmill while a continuous EKG is recorded. The treadmill speeds up according to a protocol until you reach your target heart rate (determined by your age).

Heart problems sometimes show up only when the heart is pumping hard, so by stressing the heart and monitoring the EKG, doctors can detect problems that could arise with exercise. The treadmill stress test is not perfect; most inaccuracies come from "false-positive" tests that end up being a false alarm. Other tests are more sensitive and specific to detecting heart disease, and may also be done.

SLOWLY, MAKE IT HAPPEN EVERY DAY

If you are already exercising on some days but not every day, you can take a few minutes on your days "off" to do a little exercise, so that you do something every day. You don't need to wear a heart rate monitor as long as you keep track of the time.

Getting Past the Excuses

The following suggestions will help you address common concerns that can be a barrier to exercising every day.

NO TIME TO EXERCISE

Problem-solve your schedule and plan exercise in advance. Look for blocks of time during the week when you can add in exercise. Add small bursts of physical activity to your daily routine. Do high-intensity physical activity, which takes less time to complete. Do exercises at home while the kids are playing or sleeping.

NO SUPPORT FROM FRIENDS OR FAMILY

Involve family and friends with your plans to exercise. Invite a family member or a friend for a walk. Ask them to support you in your new healthy behaviors. Plan exercise that you can do with a group or in a class.

TOO TIRED TO EXERCISE

Exercise in the morning. Plan to exercise during high-energy times of the day. Exercise anyway; most people have more energy after exercising, not less.

NOT MOTIVATED TO EXERCISE

Plan times to exercise in advance. Reward yourself for exercising. Tell friends and family about your plans to exercise, and invite them.

FEAR OF AN INJURY

Stretch, warm up, and cool down. Start slow and build on your progress.

BAD WEATHER

Always have a backup plan for exercise indoors in case of inclement weather.

TRAVEL

Walk laps around the airport. Use the hotel gym. Pack an exercise DVD to play on your laptop computer or pack a jump rope. Ask about local workout facilities or take a walk and explore new neighborhoods.

For many of my patients, getting started on a daily exercise routine was the hardest part. It just seemed so daunting and unrealistic to have a lifelong plan of exercising every day. The solution to getting started is to start slow. As I have said throughout this book, the key is to do something that is sustainable. If you aren't used to exercising and you start off too hard, you'll feel sore and tired the next day and won't want to keep exercising. Use my approach of adding positive behaviors to your life one by one, and add exercise to your life minute by minute.

If you aren't exercising every day, make your first goal to exercise for one or two minutes a day. Does that sound ridiculous? You may be thinking that it will take longer to put on your workout clothes than to exercise. You don't even need to put on workout clothes. Just wear a pair of comfortable shoes and walk around for a minute or two, being conscious that you are doing a specific, fat-burning exercise. This needs to be a minute or two in addition to all the other walking you would normally do for the day.

If you already exercise, but you don't exercise every day, take on this assignment for the days you don't exercise. If you go to the gym three days a week, make it a point to exercise for one to two minutes on the days you don't go to the gym. For even better results, do it every day, even when you do go to the gym.

Walk with a Friend

Taking a walk with a friend is one of the best forms of exercise. It is a fun way to relax and enjoy getting physical activity.

Starting a Walking Program

WEEKS	MINUTES WALKING
1 to 4	1 to 2
4 to 6	3 to 10
6 to 8	10 to 15
8 to 10	15 to 20
10 to 12	20 to 30
12 to 24	30 to 60
24+	60 to 90+

Warm Up, Stretch, and Cool Down

Take a few minutes to warm up, stretch, and cool down each time you exercise. It is an investment in your time that helps prevent injuries, which is one of the most common reasons people stop exercising. Take some time to learn how to stretch properly. Take a class or buy a DVD.

After you have established a routine of doing at least one to two minutes of mindful exercise every day, you can increase the amount of time you spend doing it. You can make a few days a week your longer days or just add a few minutes to each day. Gradually increase the time you exercise, with a goal of sixty to ninety minutes daily. Many of my patients who did this have told me that in retrospect, they wish they had been exercising their whole lives.

Get Addicted to Exercise

Even if exercising doesn't make you feel better right away, keep exercising. Many of my patients have told me that they didn't enjoy exercising for six months or longer. But eventually, when your body gets used to exercising every day, you will feel bad if you miss exercise. You might say this means you are addicted to exercise. If so, this is a good addiction to have!

PLAN AHEAD TO MAKE EXERCISE A PRIORITY

Many of my patients tell me that they don't have enough time to exercise sixty to ninety minutes every day. Yes, this is a significant amount of time. Devoting sixty to ninety minutes a day to any activity requires planning and commitment. For most people, reaching this ultimate goal does not happen by itself. Achieving the goal of exercising sixty to ninety minutes every day means that you have to make exercise a priority.

This is a commitment kept by many of my patients who have lost a lot of weight and keep it off. Most of them changed their lives to make daily exercise a top priority. If their routine changes, they plan ahead to solve any issues that might get in the way of exercising for that day. For example, one of my patients had to drive ten hours to a funeral. She stopped at rest stops along the way and took ten-to-fifteen-minute walk breaks, adding up to a full day of exercise. There are many situations that can get in the way of exercising daily. By making daily exercise a priority, you will be able to plan your daily routine as well as times when your routine changes to ensure you are able to exercise every day.

PUT ON YOUR WORKOUT CLOTHES

Jeff Galloway, a former Olympian runner, says that if you want to exercise, you have to put on your workout clothes.

Sometimes it can be very difficult to get motivated to exercise. That walk or run may not sound that appealing, and you just don't feel like working out. You know you should exercise, but you just don't have the motivation or you feel tired, or you just have other things you want to do.

Instead of worrying about the whole workout, just get dressed. Put on your workout clothes and your shoes as a first step. Don't even think about the exercise, just focus on getting dressed. Once you are dressed, walk over to your front door. Put your hand on the doorknob, open the door, and walk out. (Make sure to lock the door and bring your keys!) You still don't need to think about working out. Just walk down your driveway and start walking. Before you know it you are exercising!

The key is not to let the exercise itself make you feel overwhelmed. Approach it step by step. Just changing your clothes will help your mind refocus into the mode of exercising and it may not seem like such a difficult chore.

Do Fat-Burning Exercises

Consistent aerobic physical activity is one of the best ways to burn fat because it activates the metabolic hormones. Exercise alleviates insulin resistance and leptin resistance, which leads to long-term, sustained weight loss. Studies have shown that consistent exercise, such as walking or jogging, can be the most important factor when it comes to long-term weight maintenance.

Fat-burning exercise is something you can do for a sustained period—at least thirty minutes, but sixty minutes or longer is even better. This is moderate-intensity aerobic exercise and helps build endurance. The CDC defines moderate-intensity physical activity as breathing hard, but not too hard to talk or sing. You should be able to get your heart rate to 100 to 140 or higher, depending on your level of fitness and the activity you are doing.

Substitute Physical Activity for Exercise

Physical activity is a great substitute for planned exercise. The difference between physical activity and exercise is the purpose of the activity. The purpose of exercise is health. Physical activity is any activity that involves moving the body. Mowing the lawn, pacing the room while talking on the phone, gardening, cooking, house cleaning, walking the dog, shopping, and playing with kids are all great types of physical activity. Take time at work to intentionally get up from your desk and walk around. There are limitless forms of physical activity. The key is being more active all the time.

Consistency Is the Key

Whatever you do for exercise, the key to success is consistent frequency. I want you to make it a goal to exercise every day.

A good goal is to get approximately 350 to 450 minutes (roughly six to eight hours) of fat-burning exercise every week. If you aren't able to do this much at first, don't worry. Start doing as much as you can and slowly increase the amount of exercise using the guide above.

There are so many different types of exercise you can do. The type is not as important as the consistency. You should do different types of fat-burning exercises so that you (and your muscles) don't get bored. This also gives you different options for various circumstances, such as when it snows or when it is very hot outside.

FAT-BURNING EXERCISES

- Biking
- Boxing
- Calisthenics
- Car washing
- Carrying boxes
- Chopping wood
- Circuit weight training
- Climbing stairs
- Cross-country skiing
- Dancing
- Elliptical machine
- Fitness classes
- Hiking
- Ice skating
- Jogging
- Jumping on a trampoline or in a funhouse
- Lacrosse
- Martial arts
- Playground, active playing
- Racquetball
- Recumbent bike
- Roller skating
- Rowing or rowing machine
- Skipping
- Soccer
- Sports that require constant running or jogging
- StairMaster
- Swimming
- Treading water
- Treadmill
- Ultimate Frisbee
- Walking
- Walking in water
- Water aerobics
- Wrestling

GET PROPER SHOES FOR WALKING

Most of my patients use walking as their main type of fat-burning exercise. Many people underestimate the power of walking as an exercise, but it is by far one of the best forms of aerobic physical activity. Be sure to invest in a good pair of walking or running shoes and get new ones every 500 to 1,000 miles, or 805 to 1,600 km (check the manufacturer's instructions). I recommend getting a running shoe one-half to one size larger than your dress shoe size to protect your toes. It is good to buy your running shoes in a store with an experienced salesperson who can watch you walk or run inside the store and suggest the best shoe for you.

More vigorous exercises, such as jogging, cross-country skiing, swimming, or biking, are even better for fat burning and can reduce the time you need to spend exercising each week.

Exercise Regardless

Even if you have an injury or a disability, you should still exercise. Consistent physical activity has health benefits for everyone. Work with your doctor to find exercises that you can do on a daily basis.

Do Muscle-Building Exercises

In addition to fat-burning exercise, you should do some muscle- and strength-building exercises two, three, or more days each week. All exercise builds muscle, but resistance exercises—including isometric exercises, working with resistance bands, calisthenics (sit-ups and push-ups), yoga, gardening with shoveling, and weight training—are most effective for building muscle.

Muscle-building exercises are sometimes referred to as anaerobic exercise. They build strength, in contrast to the aerobic fat-burning exercises that also help increase cardiovascular fitness. I recommend including resistance or weight training for at least sixty minutes per week (twenty minutes, three times a week). The key is for you to be consistent. It is a good idea to rest at least one day between training sessions to let the body repair and rebuild. You don't have to spend hours in the gym, but doing muscle-building exercises for sixty minutes each week can be very effective in helping you increase your lean body mass.

Your body's lean body mass or muscle mass is one of the primary factors that determines your metabolism. By doing exercises that help you build up muscle, you can raise your metabolism, helping you burn more calories twenty-four hours a day. Having more muscle improves leptin and insulin resistance as well.

When you do any type of resistance training, your muscles contract and constrict the blood vessels running through them. When your muscles relax, a surge of blood flows through the muscles, bringing oxygen and making them stronger. Consistent resistance training, even just a small amount, will result in the strengthening and enlargement of your muscles.

A Little Weight-Room Lingo

A repetition is one complete movement of a muscle-building activity. A set is a group of repetitions. You should do sets of ten to fifteen repetitions with lighter weights instead of using heavier weights and fewer repetitions. More repetitions with lighter weight reduces your risk for injuries and has been shown to have a longer lasting effect on building muscle than doing fewer repetitions with heavier weights. Do two to four sets of each exercise. Make sure you take a minute or two to rest after each set of weights. Studies in rats have shown that insufficient rest time with high-intensity resistance exercises causes muscle loss instead of muscle growth.

Exercise in the Morning

Make an effort to exercise early in the day, especially important if you have trouble finding time to exercise, or you feel too tired to exercise, or aren't motivated to exercise. People who exercise early in the day have more energy and feel less hungry all day long.

Many of my patients have told me they aren't morning people and didn't think they could exercise in the morning. I advised them to wake up a little earlier and try it. You don't have to start out with a ninety-minute workout in the morning, but try waking up ten minutes earlier and taking a short walk.

Plan your schedule so that you can get to sleep on time the night before. Set out your workout clothes and shoes and have a detailed plan for what exercise you are going to do. As you give it a try, keep the long-term goal of making morning exercise part of your daily routine.

EARLY BIRDS ARE MORE CONSISTENT

Studies have shown that people who exercise in the morning are more likely to exercise consistently than those who exercise later in the day. When you exercise early, there are fewer barriers to prevent you from exercising. Many people start out the day with good intentions to exercise later in the day, but something gets in the way.

Indeed, as the stressors of the day add to the stress of trying healthy behaviors, your motivation to exercise slips away later in the day. This is a natural response and is similar to the reason people stress-eat. Exercising in the morning means that you have made exercise a priority in your life, and thus reduces the stress in your life.

Try Multiple Small Bouts of Exercise in One Day

Many of my patients have done well by breaking up their exercise into multiple small bouts throughout the day. This is a great way to fit in more physical activity and help make it part of your everyday routine. It doesn't matter if you walk for an hour straight or do three twenty-minute sessions; both are equally effective at burning calories and boosting metabolism.

Think ahead about the times you plan to exercise and make arrangements to ensure that you follow your plan. Some of my patients like wearing running shoes as their everyday shoes so that they can get in a short walk whenever they can.

Many of my patients don't have time to get in all their physical activity at once. Even if you break it into three or four short bursts of exercise, you will still reap the benefits. By incorporating small amounts of physical activity when you can, it will help you increase the overall amount of exercise you are doing and help your metabolism stay higher though the day.

TWO-A-DAY WORKOUTS FOR SLOW OR STALLED WEIGHT LOSS

A couple bouts of planned exercise can be a great way to boost slowed or stalled weight loss. If you have never tried exercising more than once in a day, the best way to start is on a weekend when you have more time. Make it your priority to exercise at least 90 minutes total for the day; the longer, the better. Focus on keeping your diet extra healthy on this day as well.

Make plans to incorporate more two-a-day workouts on weekends and during the week. If you exercise first thing in the morning, then you only need to find one other time to get in a workout, either at lunch or after work. Sticking to the BON! Eating Plan (see chapter 2), with regular, balanced meals, is especially important on those double workout days.

Don't Sit Too Long

You shouldn't sit down for more than one hour at a time. If you work at a desk job, take a one-minute walk break every hour. Studies have shown that sitting for more than an hour slows your metabolic rate. In fact, sitting is considered a new risk factor for heart disease. Don't sit down too long. Get up and move your body every hour.

Don't Become Undone on a Plateau

Some of my patients have told me that their weight loss slows or stalls after losing some, but not all of the weight they want to lose. They get really frustrated, because they were losing weight and feeling confident, and suddenly those same habits weren't getting them the results they saw earlier. As I've discussed throughout this book, this situation can happen for many reasons. In my experience, when weight loss slows or stalls, many people become frustrated and slowly stop doing all the healthy behaviors that it took to get them to that point. Before they know it, they have started gaining a little weight and eventually even more.

Have Fun Exercising!

Exercise is very closely linked to our brain's motivation and reward centers. If you choose an activity you enjoy doing, you are more likely to do it on a consistent basis. Even if another exercise burns more calories than the one you like, you are better off doing the one you enjoy. As I discuss in chapter 3, the same dopamine reward pathway also responds to the rewarding properties of food. When you enjoy exercising, your brain is rewarded in a way not linked to food. In other words, you can satisfy brain reward pathways by doing fun exercise instead of by eating.

Studies have shown that the camaraderie from working out with the same group of people increases your likelihood of continuing to exercise. Solo workouts, especially at the end of the day, are less likely to result in a consistent exercise pattern.

One of my patients would jog as her main form of exercise, but she hated doing it. Jogging was always a chore, but she felt like she would not burn as many calories if she walked. I suggested that she start walking with her husband instead of jogging. She was able to walk with her husband about twice as frequently as jogging by herself. The result was she ended up getting in a lot more exercise.

Many of my patients enjoy walking with their spouses because they get to talk and enjoy each other's company at the same time they are exercising. You should also seek out friends who will exercise with you. Find classes you can take with other people. Play sports or even join a league. The key is to find ways of getting physical activity doing things you love to do.

Eat a Light, Slow-Carb Snack Before You Exercise

You should never exercise when hungry because it will dampen the benefits and can result in muscle loss. Have a healthy light snack before you exercise. You don't need to eat a huge meal, but if your last meal was more than two to three hours prior, a 100- to 200-calorie snack that contains slow carbohydrates eaten fifteen to thirty minutes prior to exercise can be very helpful (e.g., a piece of fruit, some baby carrots, or some yogurt).

If you exercise when you are hungry, your body will burn muscle as fuel. If you have a light, slow-carbohydrate snack fifteen to thirty minutes before exercising, it gives your body a little fuel and allows your body to burn fat instead of muscle. This allows you to exercise for longer and have more energy when you are done. You'll build muscle instead of burning it, which raises metabolism and helps burn more fat.

Strengthen Your Neck and Chest Muscles to Activate Brown Fat

A lot of people have problems related to the muscles of the neck and upper chest. The symptoms can be neck pain, headaches, back pain, or feelings of chronic tension and stress.

You should make if a habit of stretching and exercising your neck and upper chest muscles for at least five minutes every day. These muscles control our posture. Many of our daily activities are directed toward our front, including using a computer, driving, reading, or cooking. The activities of a modern lifestyle can cause these muscles to become distorted; some get used too much, while others aren't used enough.

Deep breathing is the first step in activating and warming up the muscles of the neck and upper chest. Normal shallow breaths cause these muscles to

Listen to Upbeat Music

When doing moderate-intensity or vigorous exercise, listen to the rhythm and tempo of upbeat music and allow it to help you to speed up your pace. You should listen to music that you enjoy. Listening to upbeat music helps the time pass more quickly and distracts you from monotony.

In one of many studies, researchers assessed the effects of slow and fast tempo music with participants who were riding an exercise bike. When listening to the more upbeat music with a faster tempo, participants peddled harder and faster and produced more power with each stroke of the pedal. The participants also said they enjoyed listening to the music.

shorten and contract. Sit at the edge of a chair and place your feet firmly in front of you. Place your hands on your abdomen, drop your shoulders, and close your eyes. Take slow deep breaths, taking time to feel the rise and fall of your belly and your chest as you inhale and exhale. Do this for ten to twenty breaths at least once every day, or even better, several times each day.

Slowly warm up the muscles in your neck and upper chest by standing straight with your feet shoulders'-width apart. Roll your head from side to side in a gentle motion. Then raise your arms over your head and move them around up and down, back and forth, keeping the elbows straight or slightly bent. Put your hands behind your head, fingers interlocked, and slowly move your elbows out, stretching your upper chest. Take some time to learn other stretches and exercises for your neck and upper chest that feel good and you like to do. Try chin tucks, jumping jacks, or push-ups. Swimming is an excellent exercise for the neck and upper chest.

The idea is to do gentle stretching and exercises for your neck and upper chest for a few minutes every day, several times if possible. Take care not to strain the neck muscles, although chest exercises can be more vigorous. If you work out with a trainer, ask them to spend a little extra time on your neck and upper chest. Use a band, a medicine ball, or bench press and dumbbell fly with light weights.

ACTIVATE CALORIE-BURNING BROWN FAT

Most of the fat in our body is white fat, which produces inflammation chemicals that lead to leptin resistance, cardiovascular disease, and other health problems. Brown fat is a healthy type of metabolically active fat that burns calories and generates heat.

Until recently, it was debated whether or not humans even had brown fat. Most of what we knew about brown fat was from mice. But now we know that humans do have brown fat, most of which is located in the deep tissues of the neck and upper chest. This is the same part of the body that tends to get neglected when you don't exercise enough or if you do standard types of exercise that don't focus on the neck and upper chest. When you strengthen the muscles of the neck and upper chest, it helps to activate brown fat, which raises your metabolism and helps your body burn more calories by generating more body heat.

Exercise in the Water to Make White Fat Act Like Brown Fat

I personally enjoy swimming as a fat-burning exercise. Swimming is remarkably relaxing and an extremely good form of aerobic exercise. You can swim at your own pace, with a leisurely swim or swimming freestyle, adding in a few sprints and doing flip turns. But swimming is not the only exercise you can do in the water.

Start off slowly by walking in the water. Walk a few laps back and forth at your own pace. Try using a kickboard or a noodle. Tread water for one minute, two minutes, five, ten, and so on. Play pool volleyball, Marco Polo, water polo, or just throw a ball with a friend. Go to a water aerobics class. You don't have to be a swimmer to get in the water for physical activity.

Any type of exercise in water gives you a double advantage. Submersing yourself in water that's cooler than 98 degrees Farenheit (36.6 degrees Celsius) will pull heat from your body, forcing you to generate more body heat to keep you warm. This raises your metabolism and burns more calories. Exposing your body to the colder temperatures of a swimming pool on a regular basis will activate fat cells to generate more heat and burn more calories.

MAKE WAY FOR "BROWNISH" FAT

Cold exposure in the water or any activities, such as skiing and hiking in winter, turns white fat cells into "brownish" fat cells. Even turning down the thermostat in your home a couple of degrees can help your white fat become a little more brownish. As I discussed in the section above, most of the brown fat in our body is located in the deep tissues of our neck and upper chest.

To date, scientists have not found a way to turn white fat into brown fat. However, they have found a way to make white fat behave like brown fat. They call this brownish fat or beige fat. This good-behaving white fat also burns more calories and produces fewer harmful inflammation chemicals than regular white fat.

Unlike mice, we don't have brown fat scattered throughout our bodies. Having more brown fat is like the holy grail of fat. It just doesn't seem possible. We all wish we had more brown fat and less white fat. It would be great if scientists could find a way to give us deposits of brown fat throughout our

Wear Pool Shoes to Walk in the Pool

Buy an inexpensive pair of pool shoes so that you don't get an abrasion on the bottom of your foot. The water will soften your skin and even a few laps of walking barefoot in a pool can give you an injury if you aren't wearing pool shoes.

bodies. Even though this isn't possible, consistently exposing your body to the cold water of a swimming pool or any type of cold can make white fat behave like brown fat.

Push Yourself Longer and Harder

As you exercise on a daily basis and begin to build endurance and strength, it is important that you push out of your comfort zone by increasing the duration or the intensity of your workouts.

When you do resistance training, gradually increase the amount of weights you are using or the resistance in the machines. Continually strive to achieve higher goals, taking it to the next level. You should push yourself to the point of making new strides and new gains, but not to the point of hurting yourself or getting an injury. A little soreness the next day is okay. The soreness signifies that you are pushing your body to a new level.

Practice positive self-talk and focus on motivating yourself while you exercise. Think about how you are getting stronger and healthier. Treat each workout as an important opportunity to grow and expand. Tell yourself that anything of value takes hard work. If you want to get in better shape, you need to work for it.

STEP BY STEP

Ways to Push Past Your Comfort Zone

- Add in one to two minutes of sprints to walking, jogging, swimming, or biking.
- Walk hills instead of a flat surface, or increase the elevation on the treadmill.
- Increase your treadmill speed.
- Add five to ten minutes to your regular workout.
- Add a second workout on the weekends or your day off.
- If you take an exercise class, try to find an advanced class.
- Work out with a friend who you know will push you.
- Play a competitive sport.

DON'T REST ON YOUR LAURELS

For many people, the biggest barrier to getting regular exercise is getting started and out the door on a habitual basis. But even if you have established a regular workout routine, you should always work on increasing the intensity and the duration of your workouts. As you push yourself to do more and more, your body will respond by building more muscle and burning more fat.

CHAPTER

10

Create a Support System

Although a healthy eating plan and exercise are key to losing weight, there are many other things you can do to beat overeating permanently, from improving your "sleep hygiene" to really allowing yourself to relax. By adding these healthy behaviors and enlisting the help of your family and friends, you can build a support system that will keep you on track.

Support Yourself with Better Sleep

Healthy sleep is one of the most important things to achieve if you want to lose weight permanently. In the past twenty years, hundreds of studies have linked poor sleep to weight gain as well as a host of weight-related disorders, such as diabetes, heart disease, and sleep apnea. Having good sleep hygiene is as important as brushing your teeth. A lack of sleep has powerful effects on hunger hormones, such as leptin, ghrelin, and insulin, increasing appetite and cravings—and your ability to lose weight and keep it off.

Bad hygiene is unsanitary, and bad sleep hygiene is also unhealthy. According to the CDC, 70 million Americans have unhealthy sleep. There is a lot you can do to improve your sleep hygiene and your sleep. You should get seven to nine hours of good-quality sleep every night. Studies have shown that getting too little sleep or too much sleep can lead to weight gain and obesity.

***action*plan**

Create a Support System

- *Get better sleep.*
- *Use relaxation as a substitute.*
- *Involve family and friends.*
- *Use tools to support weight loss.*
- *Beat overeating in restaurants.*
- *Have a realistic plan for travel.*
- *Educate yourself.*
- *Get medical help.*

Having healthy sleep takes some work, just like having a healthy diet and exercising. Good sleep doesn't always come naturally. Take the time to improve your sleep hygiene as part of a total lifestyle program. Healthy sleep is just as important as eating healthy food and exercising regularly.

Many people with disrupted sleep overeat because their biological clock is out of sync with their hunger hormones. There has been a lot of research linking biological clock disturbances with slowed metabolism and increased appetite and carbohydrate cravings. One study found that sleep-deprived adults ate more than 300 calories a day more than those who were well-rested. When your body clock is out of sync, it has effects on leptin, ghrelin, insulin, and many other hormones.

THE IMPORTANCE OF BEING IN SYNC

Your circadian rhythm, or biological clock center, is in your brain. Recently, scientists have discovered that your organs—including your liver, pancreas, and bowels—all have their own independent biological clocks. When the central biologic clock in the brain gets out of sync with the body's other biological clocks, it causes hormone disruptions, such as leptin and insulin resistance, and boosts levels of the hunger hormones ghrelin, neuropeptide Y, and cortisol. The body responds with increased appetite and weight gain.

Sleep deprivation has also been shown to decrease the ability of glucose to enter brain cells. Studies have also found that sleep-deprived people have cravings for carbohydrates. Researchers believe that carbohydrate cravings are the body's way of responding to this problem with glucose not getting into brain cells.

Use the following recommendations to help your hunger hormones by improving your sleep.

EAT MEALS AND SNACKS ON A SCHEDULE

Studies have shown that eating on a schedule helps to reset the body's biologic clock and helps normalize the sleep and wake cycle.

REDUCE (OR ELIMINATE) CIGARETTES

If there isn't reason enough to quit smoking, put better sleep on the list. Smoking and other tobacco products decrease the quality of your sleep.

DON'T HAVE CAFFEINE AFTER NOON

Caffeine is a stimulant that can affect your sleep, especially if you drink it late in the day. Try to avoid that late afternoon cup of coffee as a quick energy boost. As you improve your sleep hygiene, you will have more energy in the afternoon and won't feel like you need caffeine.

RESIST TAKING NAPS

Even if you feel like you need to take a nap, don't do it. Naps make it more difficult to sleep at night, making you feel tired the next day and wanting to take another nap. Break the cycle by resisting a nap, and soon you won't need one. If you have healthy sleep hygiene and still need to take naps, you may have narcolepsy (see below).

DON'T USE YOUR BEDROOM FOR ANYTHING OTHER THAN SLEEP

Don't watch TV in your bedroom. Don't read books, pay bills, go on a computer, or eat in your room. I know this is very unpopular advice, but you have to hear it. Using your bedroom for anything other than sleep creates a distraction that can make it difficult to fall asleep or disturb your sleep.

EXERCISE, BUT NOT FOR TWO HOURS BEFORE BEDTIME

Among its other benefits, exercise helps you have more deep, restful sleep. Studies have shown that people who don't get enough sleep tend not to get enough exercise. If you feel sleepy, you won't feel motivated to exercise. Yet exercise will improve your sleep, and vice versa—healthy sleep improves muscle recovery after exercise.

AVOID (OR LIMIT) ALCOHOL, ESPECIALLY BEFORE BEDTIME

Alcohol is one of the most common causes of disturbed sleep. Many of my patients who drink a glass of wine before bedtime have told me that they fall asleep fine but they wake up at 2 or 3 a.m. and can't go back to sleep. Some patients even describe suddenly waking up with a feeling of panic or racing heart. When they stop drinking well before bedtime, the problem goes away. Wine or any alcohol makes you feel sleepy. But alcohol wears off in three or four hours so that you wake up and can't go back to sleep.

START YOUR BEDTIME RITUAL TWO HOURS IN ADVANCE

Most people don't fall asleep unless they have been home for at least two hours. Before bedtime, make a mental note that you need to start unwinding. You should be finishing dinner and getting ready to eat a sweet, slow-carbohydrate dessert like I talk about in chapter 5. Read a book, watch a television show, drink a cup of noncaffeinated tea, and just relax for a while before you go to sleep.

TURN OFF STIMULATING ACTIVITIES EARLY

Don't play video games, go on the Internet, watch stimulating television programs, or exercise two hours before bedtime. Try not to do homework (especially math) too close to bedtime.

TAKE A HOT BATH OR SHOWER BEFORE BED

This is standard advice from sleep experts because it helps you relax; studies show that it improves sleep.

GO TO BED EARLIER

For many people, the problem is simply not getting enough sleep. You need to get seven to nine hours of sleep every night. If you aren't getting enough sleep, problem-solve your schedule so that you can get to bed earlier and ensure that you will get enough sleep.

MAKE YOUR BEDROOM DARK

Use heavy curtains or shades and remove bright clocks, computer monitors, or other sources of light. Many studies have linked the sleep and awake cycle with light and dark. Melatonin is a hormone made by the pineal gland that makes you feel sleepy. Bright light, especially blue light, such as that from computer monitors (420 to 480 nm on the spectrum), and red light (630 to 700 nm on the spectrum), suppresses melatonin levels and resets your biological clock to daytime. Turn down the lights at night. Use sepia tones if you use a computer monitor. Avoid bright lights before bedtime. If you wake up in the middle of the night, don't turn on bright lights. Bright lights suppress melatonin production and reset your biologic clock to daytime. Use bright lights to help you wake up in the morning. Bright lights help tell your body that it is daytime and keep your circadian rhythm in sync.

KEEP YOUR BEDROOM QUIET

For obvious reasons, you need to have quiet to sleep. Do whatever you can to reduce or eliminate sources of noise in your bedroom. If your spouse snores, you need to come up with a plan so that the snoring doesn't disturb your sleep. Snoring can be a sign of sleep apnea; see below.

COOL DOWN YOUR BEDROOM

Your body needs to cool its core temperature when you sleep. If you sleep in warm or hot temperatures, you aren't able to have deep restful sleep because your body can't cool down. Keeping your bedroom cool may not be most energy efficient, but it does help you have great sleep.

MAKE YOUR BED AS COMFORTABLE AS POSSIBLE

Use very comfortable sheets, pillows, and most important, a good mattress. Don't cut corners on these important items. You spend a third of your life in your bed, longer than in your car. You should buy the most comfortable mattress, the best sheets, and the most comfortable pillow you can afford.

ELIMINATE DISTRACTIONS AND CLUTTER

Remove distractions, such as televisions, piles of papers or bills, books, cell phones, pets, children old enough to be sleeping in their own beds, and so on from your bedroom. Keep your bedroom clean and organized, clear out drawers in nightstands, and remove any other clutter. All these items can have an effect on your mind and distract you from falling asleep and having deep restful sleep.

Some of my patients have told me that having a clutter-free bedroom is an extremely difficult task. But I have also seen that for the ones that take on the challenge, the payoff is huge. Most of them end up cleaning and organizing their whole house. This brings a sense of freedom and relaxation. When they free themselves of all the clutter and distractions, they have deep, restful sleep.

MEDITATE AT BEDTIME

One survey found that almost 50 percent of Americans don't get enough sleep because they are too stressed or worried to sleep. Stress-induced insomnia is one of the most common forms of insomnia. You may not be able to eliminate

Tip: Freeze Your Sheets

If you are stuck in a situation where you can't get a cool bedroom, try freezing your sheets for a few hours and put them on your bed just before you go to sleep.

the stressors in your life, but you should take a few minutes to let it all go and focus on feeling peaceful and calm.

Most people know about meditation and other relaxation techniques to help them fall asleep, but they rarely actually do it. Try to clear your head of all the activities of the day and think peaceful thoughts.

TAKE SOME MELATONIN

Taking 1 to 3 mg of melatonin at bedtime can be helpful for resetting the sleep/wake cycle. Melatonin is also used to treat jet lag. There have been a lot of short-term studies on melatonin, but no long-term safety studies have been done. Use melatonin if your sleep cycle is out of sync to help reset your biological clock. I recommend using melatonin for a few days at a time, but some of my patients have benefited from using it nightly to treat insomnia.

If you plan on taking melatonin, you should discuss this with your physician first and do so under their supervision and guidance. Fatigue and depression have been reported as side effects of melatonin.

GET CHECKED FOR A SLEEP DISORDER

Sleep disorders cause disrupted sleep and are a major cause of weight gain. There have been numerous studies linking sleep disorders to increased appetite, carbohydrate cravings, weight gain, and obesity. If you have a sleep disorder, getting it treated is an important first step to beating overeating and being healthier.

If you have excessive daytime sleepiness, you could have sleep apnea, narcolepsy, or shift work disorder. If you have an Epworth Sleepiness score of 10 or above, you may have a sleep disorder and should see your physician (see questionnaire).

Do You Have Excessive Daytime Sleepiness?

The Epworth Sleepiness Scale (ESS) is a test used by doctors to determine how sleepy their patients are. It is a simple way to measure your general level of sleepiness. The questionnaire contains eight common daytime situations for which you rate your likelihood of falling asleep or dozing off on a scale of 0 to 3.

"0"	Would never doze
"1"	Slight chance of dozing
"2"	Moderate chance of dozing
"3"	High chance of dozing

SITUATION	SCORE (CIRCLE ONE)
Sitting and reading	0 – 1 – 2 – 3
Watching television	0 – 1 – 2 – 3
Sitting inactive in a public place—for example a theater or meeting	0 – 1 – 2 – 3
Lying down to rest in the afternoon when circumstances permit	0 – 1 – 2 – 3
Sitting and talking to someone	0 – 1 – 2 – 3
Sitting quietly after lunch without alcohol	0 – 1 – 2 – 3
In a car, while stopped for a few minutes in traffic	0 – 1 – 2 – 3
As a passenger in a car for an hour without a break	0 – 1 – 2 – 3
TOTAL SCORE	____________

An ESS score of 10 or more suggests that you have excessive daytime sleepiness, which may be caused by a sleep disorder. Any score of 10 or above requires evaluation by your physician.

Do You Have Sleep Apnea?

___ Are you overweight or obese?
___ Do you have a large neck size (17 inches [43 cm] or greater in men and 16 inches [41 cm] or greater in women)
___ Do you snore?
___ Do you have "pauses" in breathing or stop breathing during sleep?
___ Do you wake up gasping for air?
___ Do you have excessive fatigue?
___ Do you wake up tired and foggy-headed?
___ Do you have trouble staying awake during the day?
___ Do you have headaches in the morning?

___ Do you have restless legs?
___ Do you have difficulty concentrating?
___ Do you have a history of high blood pressure, heart disease, stroke, or diabetes?

If you answered yes to any of these questions, you should see your doctor to be evaluated for sleep apnea.

Do You Have Narcolepsy?

___ Do you have excessive daytime sleepiness?
___ Do you sleep at inappropriate times?
___ Do you take a lot of naps?
___ Do you sleep for long periods of time?
___ Is your sleep unrefreshing?
___ Have you ever had sudden loss of strength in your muscles?
___ Have you ever felt paralyzed upon falling asleep or when awakening?
___ Have you ever had hallucinations just before falling asleep, during naps, or when awakening?

If you answered yes to any of these questions, you should see your physician to be evaluated for narcolepsy.

Do You Have Shift Work Disorder?

___ Do you frequently rotate shifts or work at night?
___ Do you start your day before 4 a.m. or work later than 7 p.m.?
___ Do you feel sleepy at times when you should be awake?
___ Do you have trouble falling asleep?
___ Do you have difficulty concentrating?
___ Do you have headaches?

If you answered yes to two or more of these questions, you should see your physician to be evaluated for shift work disorder.

Use Relaxation as a Substitute

Although it is easier said than done, relaxing and eliminating stress in your life helps lower cortisol levels and alleviates leptin and insulin resistance. A wealth of clinical studies have evaluated relaxation techniques for weight loss, and many studies have found a benefit. Use relaxing activities as a substitute for eating unhealthy foods to satisfy your brain's dopamine reward system (see chapter 3). Find relaxing activities that are fun and that you can do on a consistent basis. Give yourself the time to read a book, watch a movie, or take a walk.

How Simple Is Deep Breathing?

Close your eyes and take a few slow, deep breaths. How easy was that? Do this several times every day, especially when you feel stressed out.

BECOME PASSIONATE ABOUT COOKING

If you enjoy cooking, make cooking healthy food your passion. Learn to create delicious healthy dishes that you love cooking *and* eating. Visit a local farmers' market or organic food market and explore new healthy foods. Try new healthy recipes that are fun to cook and eat, such as fajitas. Try an outdoor barbecue with vegetables and fish or chicken. Don't know how to cook it? Look it up online! There are many recipes on the Internet with pictures and easy instructions.

MAKE SURE YOU FIT IN EXERCISE

Many people don't exercise because they feel too stressed out, or as if they don't have enough time to exercise. A lot of research has shown that exercise helps reduce stress and makes you more productive so that you can get done what you need to do, in less time. Find ways of getting in more physical activity that you enjoy.

EXPLORE THE BENEFITS OF YOGA AND TAI CHI

Numerous studies show the benefits of yoga and tai chi for weight loss. Both are ancient practices for well-being. Yoga practitioners use breathing techniques, poses, and affirmations to integrate the body, mind, and spirit. Tai chi is a practice of comfortable, fluid movement of the body and breath to regulate energy. You can take a class in either, or buy a DVD, which will bring the benefits of these disciplines into your home.

DEAR GOD, WHY CAN'T I LOSE WEIGHT?

Studies have been mixed about spirituality, religion, and weight loss. Some studies have shown that using spirituality as an inspiration for losing weight can be very powerful and extremely effective. When you think of your body as a temple, you may be less likely to trash it. Another study found that very religious people are more likely to be overweight or obese. If eating unhealthy foods or having unhealthy eating patterns is part of your religious community activities, talk to your clergy person about healthy options.

Involve Your Family and Friends

Involve your family and friends in your healthy lifestyle. Ask them to support you. Tell them what you are doing and invite them to join you by eating more vegetables and fruits and exercising more. Try getting everyone to go on a family walk or have the whole family cook a healthy meal together.

It's important to be specific about how you want your family to support you. For example, if a certain food is tempting you, ask them to not eat it in front of you. Try to get your spouse on board by mentioning the benefits of a healthy lifestyle: slowing down aging, looking better, and having more energy. Tell your children about the advantages of physical fitness.

Family Meals Support a Healthy Lifestyle

A review of seventeen studies on nutrition and eating patterns published in the journal *Pediatrics* suggests that having family meals at least three times a week encourages healthy eating habits and reduces the risk of obesity. Eating five or more meals per week as a family reduces the risk of obesity in children by 25 percent; having three or more family meals per week reduces obesity risk by 12 percent.

It is thought that meals eaten together as a family provide an element of protection against disordered eating and unhealthy eating. Family meals are a sign of the family being connected, which can help children and adolescents talk about food and eating issues.

If there are people in your life who aren't completely on board, don't let them get in the way of having a healthy lifestyle. You should be aware that it is helpful, but not absolutely necessary, for others to be involved in your process.

INVITE YOUR FRIENDS TO JOIN YOU

Having a healthy lifestyle day in and day out can be difficult if you don't have the support of the people you interact with on a daily basis. When your children and spouse are unsupportive or unwilling to change their own lifestyle habits, it makes it even more difficult for you to stick with a healthy lifestyle. If your family is eating unhealthy food in front of you or leaving the wrappers around, it can do a lot to sabotage your good intentions. Most loved ones want to be supportive, and they may not realize that what they do has an impact on you.

Family and friends have a very powerful influence on your weight. A study published in the *New England Journal of Medicine* found that having a close friend who is overweight is a greater risk factor for your being overweight than having an overweight family member. Involving family and friends in your healthy lifestyle helps to create a supportive environment for everyone.

STEP BY STEP

New Ways to Socialize

Be honest with your friends and try to plan outings that don't involve eating unhealthy food. For example, if you normally go to a bar and have a drink with a friend, invite him or her to go for a walk instead. Team up with a friend or coworker to be your weight-loss buddy. Ask someone you know who has been successful losing weight to be your coach or mentor.

Use Tools to Support Weight Loss

If you've ever tried to keep a food diary and gave up because it was too difficult, here's a good reason to give it another go: A study published in *American Journal of Preventive Medicine* showed that keeping a food diary doubles the amount of weight lost over a five-month period.

Keeping a food diary helps you be aware of the food you eat. It allows you to see what you are doing so that you can be accountable to yourself. Using a food diary has also been shown to be an effective tool to help you keep the weight off.

Other tools, such as social networks or a blog to involve family and friends in your goal, or surfing websites for tips, recipes, and inspiration, can also provide you with fun, relaxing activities to support your weight loss.

LET YOUR FOOD DIARY INFORM YOU

Write down everything you eat, good or bad, in a food diary. Buy a small notebook and short pencil that you can keep in a pocket or pocketbook. You can keep a detailed food diary, recording each calorie you consume, or just jot down the food that you are eating. The point is to have a record of all the food you eat. Review your food diary often, so that you can transfer the written record back into your conscious thinking.

GIVE AND TAKE ON SOCIAL NETWORKS

Think of social networking as an interactive way of journaling. Social networking on Facebook, Twitter, YouTube, or a site specifically dedicated to connecting with people who are working on weight loss is a great way to enhance your communication, involve others, and get a lot of support.

When you use social networking, you also get an opportunity to help other people with their weight-loss goals and challenges. Upload a photo of your healthy meal or tweet about the great exercise you just did. Use social network sites to tell everyone about your goals and your progress.

START A WEIGHT-LOSS BLOG

Some of my patients have found it very helpful to keep a blog documenting their weight-loss journey. Making your goals and achievements public will make it more likely that you will achieve them. Blog about your weigh-ins, recipes you like, struggles, and successes. Tell all your friends and family about your blog so that you can develop a community of followers and supporters.

Weight-Loss Websites

A lot of websites connect people interested in fitness or weight loss. You can also use these sites to research recipes and lifestyle tips:

- **WebMD** (www.webmd.com/diet) contains a lot of information on fitness and healthy eating, including recipes and healthy eating guides for specific medical conditions. The site also contains an exercise and calorie calculator, a food and fitness planner, and links to the WebMD diet community, a social networking forum hosted by diet experts.
- **Eating Well** (www.eatingwell.com), **Shape** (www.shape.com), **Prevention** (www.prevention.com), **Health** (www.health.com), and **Cooking Light** (www.cookinglight.com) are the websites for the magazines by the same names. These sites have a wealth of recipes and articles on fitness, healthy eating, and healthy cooking.
- **Nutrition.gov** (www.nutrition.gov) is a site sponsored by the U.S. Department of Agriculture that features recipes, articles, and information on shopping, cooking, and meal planning.
- **Centers for Disease Control and Prevention** (www.cdc.gov/healthyweight) is a site with articles, videos, and podcasts about healthy eating and weight loss.
- **Fruits and Vegetables Matter** (www.fruitsandveggiesmatter.gov) is another website sponsored by the CDC that highlights fruits and vegetables with tips, recipes, and tools.
- **Joy Bauer** (www.joybauer.com) *Today* show expert Joy Bauer has developed a site that allows you to create a customized diet plan. The site has a lot of weight-loss tools and inspirational success stories.
- **Jillian Michaels** (www.jillianmichaels.com), a former trainer on TV's *The Biggest Loser*, features weight-loss and fitness information, podcasts, blogs, and success stories, along with recipes and tools.
- **Calorie King** (www.calorieking.com) contains nutritional information for thousands of foods, including restaurant foods.
- **My Fitness Pal** (www.myfitnesspal.com) is a site with an online food and exercise diary, weight-loss blogs, and community forums.

Just Say No to Appetizers

Many diet experts recommend substituting an appetizer for an entrée at a restaurant to save calories, but I disagree. Most appetizers do what they are supposed to do and stimulate your appetite. Appetizers tend to be high-calorie, low-volume foods, and are frequently fried. Instead, choose a healthier entrée.

Beat Overeating in Restaurants

Long-term, sustained weight loss is difficult when you eat in a lot of restaurants. My advice is to limit restaurant meals to once a week. You don't have to avoid restaurants completely, but make it a special event. Think of your meal in a restaurant as a reward for a week of healthy eating and consistent exercise.

It is a challenge to eat healthy foods in restaurants. The typical restaurant meal contains 60 percent more calories than a home-cooked meal. Most restaurant menus have healthy choices, but we don't always want to pick the healthiest thing on the menu. Studies have shown that people who eat frequently in restaurants tend to weigh more.

STEP BY STEP

Ways to Beat Overeating in Restaurants

- Order a side order of extra vegetables.
- Order first, so other people don't tempt you to order less-healthy food.
- Ask for half of your meal to be wrapped in a to-go box before it is brought to the table.
- Share an entrée.
- Have a salad before your meal.
- Substitute fruit or vegetables for fries.
- Request that items be prepared without butter or oil.
- Order salad dressing, gravy, and sauces on the side and only use a small amount.
- Drink water instead of beverages with calories.
- Avoid all-you-can-eat buffets.
- Ask the waiter not to bring bread to the table.
- Choose broiled, grilled, poached, steamed, roasted, or baked instead of fried or sautéed.
- Choose marinara over cream sauce.
- Choose broth-based soups over cream soups.
- Don't be afraid to make a special order; restaurants are in business to serve you.

Be conscious of the food you eat in a restaurant. Restaurant portions are typically double or triple a normal-size portion. Don't just assume a food is healthy, because chances are that any food prepared in a restaurant has more calories than you realize. Focus on eating larger portions of low-calorie foods early in the meal and eat smaller portions of high-calorie foods later in the meal.

Have a Realistic Plan for Travel

When you travel, eating healthy food and getting enough exercise can be especially challenging. Many of my patients have learned how to travel for business or pleasure and still eat healthy foods. Airports, hotels, and convention centers are starting to offer healthy options.

When I go to endocrine conferences, I bring my own healthy food in a brown bag lunch because there is always a long line for the food and I don't want to miss the next talk. I have learned that if I don't bring my own food, I'll end up eating the unhealthy snacks they have in the exhibit hall.

Wherever you go or whatever you do, try not to let it get you too far off track. Make an effort to add in some healthy foods or exercise on your trip to help prevent weight gain when you travel.

STEP BY STEP

Ways to Stay Healthy When You Travel

- Pack a cooler of healthy snacks, such as fresh fruit, cut-up raw vegetables, or yogurt.
- Pack a water bottle to fill up in the airport.
- Research healthy restaurant options before you go.
- Bring your workout clothes and shoes.
- Ask the hotel for directions to a nearby grocery store.
- Use the hotel gym.
- Wear running shoes when you travel and walk extra laps in the terminal while waiting for your plane.
- Do not eat the peanuts or cookies on the plane.
- Bring your own food on the plane so you won't eat the snack foods offered.
- Ask room service to prepare a healthy "brown bag" lunch for you.

Understand a Restaurant's Motivation

Studies show that people rate restaurants more highly if they serve large portions than for the quality of the food. Restaurants want you to enjoy the experience at their restaurant. Most restaurant food has a lot more calories than homemade food, which is no big secret. But most people don't know how many calories they are eating, which can be hundreds more than they realized. The point is that restaurants don't want to broadcast the nutritional content of their food. They want you to enjoy their food so you will come back to the restaurant. By being aware of this, you can make better decisions and be more conscious about the foods that you are eating.

Get Medical Help

You should get regular checkups from your physician. If you are eating a healthy balanced diet and getting regular exercise and you are still not losing weight, you could have a medical condition or a hormonal imbalance that is interfering with weight loss. If your hormones are out of whack, you may not lose weight even with a healthy eating plan.

Many medications, such as those used to treat diabetes, high blood pressure, chronic pain, anxiety, and depression, can have weight gain as a side effect. Review your medications with your doctor to see if any of them might be causing you to hold on to excess weight. It is still possible to lose weight if you have to take these medications, but you'll need to work a little harder to overcome the effect.

MEDICATIONS THAT CAN MAKE YOU GAIN WEIGHT

- Antihistamines (diphenhydramine)
- Antipsychotics
  (chlorpromazine, haloperidol, olanzapine, risperidone, quetiapine)
- Beta-blockers (atenolol, metoprolol, propranolol, nadolol)
- Corticosteroids
  (prednisone, dexamethasone, hydrocortisone, prednisolone)
- Gabapentin
- High-dose birth control pills that contain 50 mcg ethinyl estradiol (Ortho-Novum 1/50, Ovral, Ogestrel, Demulen 1/50, Ovcon 50, Zovia 1/50)
- Insulin
- Lithium
- SSRI antidepressant/antianxiety (mirtazapine, fluoxetine, sertraline, citalopram, escitalopram, paroxetine)
- Sulfonylureas (glipizide, glyburide, glimepiride)
- Thiazolidinediones (rosiglitazone, pioglitazone)
- Tricyclic antidepressants
  (amitriptyline, desipramine, imipramine, nortriptyline)
- Valproate

CONSIDER A MEDICAL WEIGHT-LOSS PROGRAM

As a weight-loss specialist, I've worked with a lot of patients in our medical weight-loss program in partnership with Health Management Resources Corporation (HMR). Many of the patients in our program have lost more than 100 pounds (45 kg). This program and other medical weight-loss programs require attendance in a weekly class and uses medical weight-loss foods, such as shakes and entrées, that help patients lose a lot of weight rapidly and safely.

Medical weight-loss programs are helpful if you have a lot of weight to lose or if you have trouble doing it on your own. The key to being successful with a medical weight-loss program is strict adherence to your eating plan and exercise prescription. Studies have shown that when patients lose a lot of weight in the early phases of a medical weight-loss program, it motivates them to stick with the program, and they end up losing more weight and are better at keeping it off. A quality medical weight-loss program will provide a plan for the transition off medical weight-loss foods to a long-term weight maintenance program.

Educate Yourself

Throughout this book, I have discussed many medical conditions that can lead to hormonal imbalance and weight gain. If you have a medical condition, take time to learn about it. If you have symptoms, and don't know what is causing them, reliable health information websites can help you understand where your symptoms may be coming from, what else to look for, and how to better communicate these symptoms to your doctor.

There can be a lot of misleading information on the Internet, so it is important to use reliable websites. Quackwatch (www.quackwatch.com) is a nonprofit company that exposes health-related "frauds, myths, fads, and fallacies." Their website contains up-to-date, well-researched information on the medical practices and advertising deemed dubious or obvious "quackery."

RECOMMENDED HEALTH INFORMATION WEBSITES

- Aetna Intelihealth (www.intelihealth.com)
- American Academy of Family Physicians (www.familydoctor.org)
- American Academy of Pediatrics (www.aap.org)
- American Association of Retired Persons (www.aarp.org/health)
- American Diabetes Association (www.diabetes.org)
- American Heart Association (www.heart.org)
- Asthma and Allergy Foundation of America (www.aafa.org)
- The Cleveland Clinic (http://my.clevelandclinic.org/health)
- eMedicine Health (www.emedicinehealth.com)
- Hormone Foundation (www.hormone.org)
- Mayo Clinic (www.mayoclinic.com)
- MedlinePlus (www.nlm.nih.gov/medlineplus)
- National Cancer Institute (www.cancer.gov)
- National Digestive Diseases Information Clearinghouse (www.digestive.niddk.nih.gov)
- National Heart, Lung, and Blood Institute (www.nhlbi.nih.gov)
- National Institute on Aging (www.nia.nih.gov)
- National Institutes of Health (http://health.nih.gov)
- U.S. Department of Health and Human Services (www.healthfinder.gov)
- WebMD (www.webmd.com)

CHAPTER 11

Conquer Mindless Eating

Most people eat more than they are conscious of, and don't even realize how many calories they are consuming. Even professional dietitians underestimate the number of calories they consume.

The environment we live in encourages people to eat more calories and to exercise less. You must be aware of this situation and take an active approach to fight it.

Even if you outsmart your hunger hormones, mindless eating can creep in to sabotage you. To truly beat overeating, you have to conquer mindless eating. There are lots of ways to do it; the key is finding strategies that work for you.

Inside Mindless Eating

Mindless eating is the eating we do for reasons other than hunger. The sight and smell of food can make you eat mindlessly in part because of effects on hunger hormones, such as leptin, ghrelin, and neuropeptide Y. The body and brain can be tricked into eating more calories than we realize because of subtle ways food is presented. Plates, bowls, packages, containers, labels, colors, smells, shapes, and names of products all influence how many calories we consume. We also eat mindlessly when we stress-eat or eat for boredom, anxiety, or for no apparent reason at all.

*action*plan

Stop Eating Mindlessly

- *Think about your food when you are eating.*
- *Read labels to understand portion size.*
- *Avoid hidden calories.*
- *Be aware of calories in everything you eat.*
- *Use a 9½- to 10-inch (24 to 25 cm) plate.*
- *Serve extra vegetables and fruit family style.*
- *Understand a restaurant's motivation.*
- *Make unhealthy foods difficult to access.*
- *Plan for situations that may trigger mindless eating.*
- *Be realistic about stress eating and emotional eating.*

A Nation of Mindless Eaters

Brian Wansink, Ph.D., Cornell University professor and director of the Cornell Food and Brand Lab, writes about food psychology in his book *Mindless Eating: Why We Eat More Than We Think*. "Regardless of how tuned in we believe we are to what we eat and how much we eat, we are really a nation of mindless eaters," says Wansink. His book highlights research on influences of the food environment on what, how much, and when we eat. It also shows how different factors in our environment can make us eat less or more—not because we are hungry, but because of unconscious cues manipulated by the packaged food and restaurant industry. Wansink's research was conducted in food labs, movie theaters, restaurants, homes, and shopping malls.

FIGURE THAT YOU'RE UNDERESTIMATING CALORIES

It can be very difficult to know what and how much you are eating. Even though the nutritional information is on the label, most people don't measure exact portion sizes. Restaurants often publish nutritional information about their dishes, but they can be extremely inaccurate; often, dishes contain hundreds more calories than they claim to. The reality is that the caloric content of a restaurant food is determined by the person cooking it. The cook will tend to add more butter and oil or other fattening flavorings to the dish to make it taste better.

A good rule of thumb is that even if you know a lot about nutrition and read a lot of labels, you are probably underestimating your daily calories by 20 to 25 percent. When counting calories, you should add 20 to 25 percent to account for this difference. For example, if your estimated daily calories equal 1,200, add 25 percent (300) to come up with your actual daily calories of 1,500.

Do You Eat Mindlessly?

___ Do you keep eating when you are full, even when eating something you don't love?
___ Do you overeat at all-you-can-eat buffets?
___ Do you take a second helping because it is sitting in front of you, even if you feel full?
___ Do you overeat at parties and celebrations?
___ Do you eat out of a bag or a box?
___ Are you influenced by advertisements for food?
___ Do sights and smells make you want to eat certain foods?
___ Does just going to the movie theater make you want to eat popcorn?
___ Do you overeat to celebrate special occasions?
___ Do you stress-eat or are you an emotional eater?
___ Do your thoughts wander while you are eating?
___ Do you eat in front of the TV, at the computer, or at your desk?
___ Do you snack without paying attention to what you are eating?
___ Do you eat too quickly?

If you answered yes to any of these questions, there are times that you are eating mindlessly.

Think About Your Food When Eating It

You must be conscious of the food you are eating. Savor and enjoy your food as you eat it. Don't eat meals in front of the TV or the computer, while reading, at your desk, or while driving. Take the time to think about every bite as you are eating it. When you are deep in conversation at a meal, take time so that the conversation doesn't distract you from being conscious of the food you are eating.

Studies have shown that being conscious of the food you eat can be an effective way to lose weight without being on a formal diet. Just having the awareness of what you are eating helps you regulate what you consume.

Read Labels to Understand Portion Size

You don't need to weigh and measure everything you eat, but you should know what you are eating and have a realistic idea of how many calories it contains. It is really important that you read all the labels of foods that you eat and understand what constitutes a portion size.

Labels can be deceptive, showing an incredibly small portion size to make the nutritional value look fine. But if you eat a normal amount of the food, it may actually be several portions, doubling or tripling the calories you are consuming. If you don't read the label, you are likely eating much more than you realized.

Also, don't be fooled by health claims on labels. Foods labeled *sugar free* or *fat free* can still have a lot of calories. Foods labeled *natural* or *organic* can also be very high in calories. We tend to be influenced by the way foods are labeled and packaged, and you may eat more of an item if you perceive it to be healthier or lower in calories.

Avoid Hidden Calories

Many foods that seem like they might be low in calories have more calories than you might think. When you use butter sprays and nonstick sprays, be very judicious with the amount you use. A small amount is fine, but using more than a few sprays per day can add hundreds of calories and pack on the pounds.

Butter flavor sprays (like Parkay spray and I Can't Believe It's Not Butter spray) are labeled as having zero calories per spray. There is a loophole in the labeling, which allows the product to claim it has zero calories when it actually is a high-calorie product. A single spray has 0.8 calories and 0.085 grams of fat per spray.

Those sprays really add up. Twenty-five sprays, the equivalent of 1 teaspoon, adds up to 20 calories. A typical bottle of zero-calorie butter spray has 832 calories and 93 grams of fat. A similar problem exists with nonstick cooking sprays such as Pam. They have 7 calories per one-second spray. This can add up to hundreds of extra calories as well.

Slow Down Your Meals

Eating slowly gives you more time to think about the food when you are eating it. Set down your fork and take a sip of water between bites or just take a pause in eating every once in a while. In chapter 6, I talk about how eating slowly also allows time for gut hormones, such as ghrelin and PYY, to kick in, helping you feel full and satisfied.

Think of Butter Spray as Extra Fat

In one case, my patient was following her diet very closely but wasn't losing nearly the weight she should have been. She swore she was doing everything right, exercising every day and even eating vegetables . . . something she had never done before. To make the vegetables taste better, she used "zero-calorie" butter spray. It turned out that she was using three bottles each week, giving her about 2,500 extra hidden calories. She quit using the spray and started losing weight.

Be Aware of Calories in Everything You Eat

Many people just nibble small bites of food and never take the time to think about how these calories quickly add up. When we have a small bite of food, such as an after-dinner mint, a sample at a store, or a bite from a friend's meal, we usually don't consider the calories in these items. Just a spoonful of a condiment can contain dozens of extra calories. The consumption of these foods tends to slip our minds when we recall the food we ate for the day.

Calorie Counts for Small Bites and Condiments

CONDIMENTS	
Ketchup, 1 tablespoon (15 g)	15 calories
Half-and-half, 1 small container	20 calories
Pat of butter	40 calories
Sugar cube	10 calories
Mayonnaise, 1 tablespoon (14 g)	100 calories
Olive oil, 1 tablespoon (15 ml)	80 calories
Cheese, 1-inch (2.5 cm) cube	60 calories
Parmesan cheese, 1 tablespoon (5 g)	22 calories
Sour cream, 1 tablespoon (15 g)	26 calories

(cont. next page)

Calorie Counts for Small Bites and Condiments *(cont.)*

LITTLE BITES	
10 M&M'S	34 calories
1 after-dinner mint	30 calories
1 cookie, 2-inch (5 cm) diameter	45 calories
¼ multigrain roll (0.8 oz, or 23 g)	60 calories
¼ hot dog and bun	140 calories
1 chicken tender	100 calories
10 peanuts	60 calories
10 oyster crackers	40 calories
1 cough drop	15 calories
½ of a 3-inch (7.5 cm) doughnut	95 calories
1 ounce (28 g) of trail mix	130 calories

Use a 9½- to 10-inch Plate

Many nutrition experts recommend using a plate that is about 9½ to 10 inches (24 to 25 cm) in diameter, smaller than today's standard dinner plate but not noticeably different. Your mind perceives a full plate with less food in the same way a larger plate is filled with food. If you use a large plate, a normal portion of food looks tiny.

However, studies have shown that using a plate that is too small will cause you to feel deprived, and you'll likely go back for a second helping.

Use a tall, narrow glass instead of a short wide glass. People perceive more liquid in a tall slender glass because our brain focuses more on height than width.

Serve Extra Fruits and Veggies Family Style

Always serve individual portions of proteins and grains on your plate, but allow yourself to mindlessly eat healthy foods. Bring large serving bowls to the table filled with vegetables, salad, and cut-up fruit to serve family style. When

Never Eat Chips out of a Bag

If you must eat chips, take a small portion and put them in a bowl. Never eat from a bag. Research shows that the bigger the bag, the more you will eat. People typically eat 25 to 50 percent more if a food is served in a large container.

In chapter 3, I talk about potato chips and snack foods, and how they can trigger overeating by stimulating your appetite and cravings. But when you eat chips out of a large bag, it adds mindless eating to this problem. The bigger the bag, the more chips you will eat. The same is true for popcorn. The larger the container, the more popcorn you will eat.

Fill Trays with Crunchy Veggies and Fruits

Many of my successful patients have told me that they buy larger containers of fruits and vegetables, such as baby carrots, celery, sliced apples, pea pods, and strawberries at the wholesale clubs. They fill a large container with healthy fruits and vegetables, and mindlessly nibble on it all day. This is a great way to eat a lot of extra fruits and vegetables all day long.

bowls of food sit right in front of you on a table, you are likely to mindlessly eat more.

You get to choose which items are brought out to the table and which ones are served from the kitchen. Encourage yourself and the others who are dining with you to have extra helpings of the dishes on the table.

Make Unhealthy Foods Difficult to Access

You've heard the expression: out of sight, out of mind. The best thing you can do is keep unhealthy foods out of your house. If you must keep unhealthy foods around the house, make them difficult to access—maybe at the back of your refrigerator or freezer. If you make it a little more difficult to get to something, it makes you less likely to eat it. For example, if you keep an indulgence food in your house, keep it wrapped up on a top shelf of the pantry, not out on the counter.

CONVERSELY, MAKE HEALTHY FOODS ACCESSIBLE

You'll succeed if you keep healthy foods around all the time. Fill your house with fruits, vegetables, and healthy snacks. Don't stash fruits and vegetables in a refrigerator drawer. Put them front and center on a shelf at eye level so you are tempted to eat them all the time.

Follow the same rules at the office: Don't keep unhealthy foods around. Don't put out candy, even if it is for customers. Keep lots of healthy food at work so you have something healthy to eat whenever you need it.

Plan for Situations That May Trigger Mindless Eating

In my experience, the most common situation in which people eat mindlessly is at a funeral. I have seen many patients who were doing well on their program get totally derailed by the death of a friend or loved one. Food served during these times is almost always consumed mindlessly without thinking about what is being eaten.

Likewise, happy occasions, such as celebrations, weddings, holidays, and family gatherings, are all filled with mindless eating. You shouldn't avoid funerals or celebrations, but do take some time to understand that these situations can trigger mindless eating and make a plan for them. In chapter 6, I discuss strategies for beating overeating at social events.

Be Realistic about Stress Eating and Emotional Eating

Stress eating and emotional eating come from situations, not hunger. The eating provides comfort and satisfies dopamine pleasure-and-reward pathways in the brain. People who stress-eat and eat for emotional reasons don't want to eat healthy foods. They typically eat snack foods or sweets.

When you stress-eat, it is very unlikely you are mindful of the food you are eating. The food provides comfort and relieves feelings of anxiety and depression. The only way to stop stress-eating is to deal with the stress in your life. A stress-free life is impossible, but if stress is making you overeat, then you have an excessive amount of stress.

Don't Be Tempted by All-You-Can-Eat Buffets

For obvious reasons, all-you-can-eat buffets are horrible for you. They create a situation in which you will overeat mindlessly. It's not just that there's so much food available, but that most people feel as if they need to eat a lot to get their money's worth.

STEP BY STEP

Ways to Beat Stress

- Write down all the stressors in your life on a piece of paper.
- Think about ways to address each stressor one by one.
- Learn ways to relax with meditation or deep breathing.
- Consider seeking help from a counselor or psychologist.
- Exercise daily.

Are You a Compulsive Overeater?

___ Do you binge eat?

___ Do you overeat to the point of feeling uncomfortably full at least once a week?

___ Do you feel guilty after overeating?

If you answered yes to any of these questions, you may be a compulsive overeater or have Binge Eating Disorder, and you should seek help from a physician or professional counselor.

Resources

Chapter 1 Resources

Abraham, C., and P. Sheeran. "Acting on intentions: the role of anticipated regret." *Br. J. Soc. Psychol.* 42 (2003): 495–511.

Abraham, C., and P. Sheeran. "Deciding to exercise: the role of anticipated regret." *Br. J. Health Psychol.* 9 (2004): 269–78.

Adriaanse, M. A., D. T. de Ridder, and J. B. de Wit. "Finding the critical cue: implementation intentions to change one's diet work best when tailored to personally relevant reasons for unhealthy eating." *Pers. Soc. Psychol. Bull.* 35 (2009): 60–71.

Adriaanse, M. A., et al. "Breaking habits with implementation intentions: a test of underlying processes." *Pers. Soc. Psychol. Bull.* 37 (2011): 502–13.

Adriaanse, M. A., et al. "Planning what not to eat: ironic effects of implementation intentions negating unhealthy habits." *Pers. Soc. Psychol. Bull.* 37 (2011): 69–81.

Alemi, F., et al. "Continuous self-improvement: systems thinking in a personal context." *Jt. Comm. J. Qual. Improv.* 26 (2000): 74–86.

Alemi, F., L. Pawloski, and W. F. Fallon Jr. "System thinking in a personal context to improve eating behaviors." *J. Healthc. Qual.* 25 (2003): 20–25.

Anderson-Bill, E. S., et al. "Aging and the social cognitive determinants of physical activity behavior and behavior change: evidence from the guide to health trial." *J. Aging Res.*, 2011: 505928.

Bacon, L., and L. Aphramor. "Weight science: evaluating the evidence for a paradigm shift." *Nutr. J.* 10 (2011): 9.

Bacon, L., et al. "Evaluating a 'non-diet' wellness intervention for improvement of metabolic fitness, psychological well-being and eating and activity behaviors." *Int. J. Obes. Relat. Metab. Disord.* 26 (2002): 854–65.

Bacon, L., et al. "Size acceptance and intuitive eating improve health for obese, female chronic dieters." *J. Am. Diet Assoc.* 105 (2005): 929–36.

Barkeling, B., et al., "Characterization of obese individuals who claim to detect no relationship between their eating pattern and sensations of hunger or fullness." *Int. J. Obes.* (Lond.) 31 (2007): 435–39.

Bray, G. A. "Obesity: maintenance of weight loss: setting our goals higher." *Nat. Rev. Endocrinol.* 6 (2010): 657–58.

Brickell, T. A., N. L. Chatzisarantis, and G. M. Pretty. "Using past behaviour and spontaneous implementation intentions to enhance the utility of the theory of planned behaviour in predicting exercise." *Br. J. Health Psychol.* 11 (2006): 249–62.

Conradt, M., et al. "A consultation with genetic information about obesity decreases self-blame about eating and leads to realistic weight loss goals in obese individuals." *J. Psychosom. Res.* 66 (2009): 287–95.

Conradt, M., et al. "Development of the Weight- and Body-Related Shame and Guilt scale (WEB-SG) in a nonclinical sample of obese individuals." *J. Pers. Assess.* 88 (2007): 317–27.

Conradt, M., et al. "Who copes well? Obesity-related coping and its associations with shame, guilt, and weight loss." *J. Clin. Psychol.* 64 (2008): 1129–44.

Costain, L., and H. Croker. "Helping individuals to help themselves." *Proc. Nutr. Soc.* 64 (2005): 89–96.

Edmiston, F. G., and D. R. Wagner. "Comparison of methods for setting weight loss goals in males." *Fam. Med.* 42 (2010): 575–76.

Elfhag, K., and S. Rössner. "Who succeeds in maintaining weight loss? A conceptual review of factors associated with weight loss maintenance and weight regain." *Obes. Rev.* 6 (2005): 67–85.

Freund, A. M., and M. Hennecke. "Changing eating behaviour vs. losing weight: the role of goal focus for weight loss in overweight women." *Psychol. Health*, 2011 Jul 7.

Hainer, V., H. Toplak, and A. Mitrakou. "Treatment modalities of obesity: what fits whom?" *Diabetes Care* 31 (2008): S269–77.

Hennecke, M., and A. M. Freund. "Staying on and getting back on the wagon: age-related improvement in self-regulation during a low-calorie diet." *Psychol. Aging* 25 (2010): 876–85.

Hindle, L., and C. Carpenter. "An exploration of the experiences and perceptions of people who have maintained weight loss." *J. Hum. Nutr. Diet.* 24 (2011), doi:10.1111/j.1365-277X.2011.01156.x.

Kelsey, K. S., et al. "Obesity, hope, and health: findings from the HOPE Works Community Survey." *J. Community Health*, 2011 Mar 10.

Lally, P., et al. "Experiences of habit formation: a qualitative study." *Psychol. Health Med.* 16 (2011): 484–89.

Leahey, T. M., et al. "A randomized trial testing a contingency-based weight loss intervention involving social reinforcement." *Obesity* (Silver Spring), 2011 May 19.

Lowe, M. R., and T. V. Kral. "Stress-induced eating in restrained eaters may not be caused by stress or restraint." *Appetite* 46 (2006): 16–21.

McInnis, K. J. "Diet, exercise, and the challenge of combating obesity in primary care." *J. Cardiovasc. Nurs.* 18 (2003): 93–100.

Mouttapa, M., et al. "The personal nutrition planner: a 5-week, computer-tailored intervention for women." *J. Nutr. Educ. Behav.* 43 (2011): 165–72.

Nelissen, R. M., E. de Vet, and M. Zeelenberg. "Anticipated emotions and effort allocation in weight goal striving." *Br. J. Health Psychol.* 16 (2011), doi:10.1348/135910710X494952.

Orbell, S., and B. Verplanken. "The automatic component of habit in health behavior: habit as cue-contingent automaticity." *Health Psychol.* 29 (2010): 374–83.

Palmeira, A. L., et al. "Predicting short-term weight loss using four leading health behavior change theories." *Int. J. Behav. Nutr. Phys. Act.* 4 (2007): 14.

Paxman, J. R., et al. "Weight loss is coupled with improvements to affective state in obese participants engaged in behavior change therapy based on incremental, self-selected 'small changes.'" *Nutr. Res.* 31 (2011): 327–37.

Payne, N., F. Jones, and P. R. Harris. "The role of perceived need within the theory of planned behaviour: a comparison of exercise and healthy eating." *Br. J. Health Psychol.* 9 (2004): 489–504.

Penny, S., and J. Carryer. "Obesity and health—new perspectives from bioscience research suggest directions for clinical practice." *NZ Med. J.* 124 (2011): 73–82.

Perugini, M., and R. P. Bagozzi. "The role of desires and anticipated emotions in goal-directed behaviours: broadening and deepening the theory of planned behaviour." *Br. J. Soc. Psychol.* 40 (2001): 79–98.

Rief, W., et al. "Is information on genetic determinants of obesity helpful or harmful for obese people?—A randomized clinical trial." *J. Gen. Intern Med.* 22 (2007): 1553–59.

Sullivan, H. W., and A. J. Rothman. "When planning is needed: implementation intentions and attainment of approach versus avoidance health goals." *Health Psychol.* 27 (2008): 438–44.

Tam, L., R. P. Bagozzi, and J. Spanjol. "When planning is not enough: the self-regulatory effect of implementation intentions on changing snacking habits." *Health Psychol.* 29 (2010): 284–92.

Teixeira, P. J., et al. "A review of psychosocial pre-treatment predictors of weight control." *Obes. Rev.* 6 (2005): 43–65.

Teixeira, P. J., et al. "Pretreatment predictors of attrition and successful weight management in women." *Int. J. Obes. Relat. Metab. Disord.* 28 (2004): 1124–33.

Teixeira, P. J., et al. "Who will lose weight? A reexamination of predictors of weight loss in women." *Int. J. Behav. Nutr. Phys. Act.* 1 (2004): 12.

Urbszat, D., C. P. Herman, and J. Polivy. "Eat, drink, and be merry, for tomorrow we diet: effects of anticipated deprivation on food intake in restrained and unrestrained eaters." *J. Abnorm. Psychol.* 111 (2002): 396–401.

Webb, T. L., P. Sheeran, and A. Luszczynska. "Planning to break unwanted habits: habit strength moderates implementation intention effects on behaviour change." *Br. J. Soc. Psychol.* 48 (2009): 507–23.

Whitlock, E. P., et al. "Screening and interventions for childhood overweight: a summary of evidence for the US Preventive Services Task Force." *Pediatrics* 116 (2005): E125–44.

Wing, R. R., and S. Phelan. "Long-term weight loss maintenance." *Am. J. Clin. Nutr.* 82 (2005): S222–25.

Wisotsky, W., and C. Swencionis. "Cognitive-behavioral approaches in the management of obesity." *Adolesc. Med.* 14 (2003): 37–48.

Wong, C. L., and B. A. Mullan. "Predicting breakfast consumption: an application of the theory of planned behaviour and the investigation of past behaviour and executive function." *Br. J. Health Psychol.* 14 (2009): 489–504.

Chapter 2 Resources

Agostoni, C., et al. "Role of dietary factors and food habits in the development of childhood obesity: a commentary by the ESPGHAN Committee on Nutrition." *J. Pediatr. Gastroenterol. Nutr.* 52 (2011): 662–69.

Anderson, J. W., S. B. Conley, and A. S. Nicholas. "One hundred pound weight losses with an intensive behavioral program: changes in risk factors in 118 patients with long-term follow-up." *Am. J. Clin. Nutr.* 86 (2007): 301–07.

Anderson, J. W., et al. "Health benefits of dietary fiber." *Nutr. Rev.* 67 (2009): 188–205.

Anderson, J. W., et al. "Soy compared to casein meal replacement shakes with energy-restricted diets for obese women: randomized controlled trial." *Metabolism* 56 (2007): 280–88.

Anderson, J. W., et al. "Weight loss and long-term follow-up of severely obese individuals treated with an intense behavioral program." *Int. J. Obes.* (Lond.) 31 (2007): 488–93.

Anderson, J. W., et al. "Long-term weight-loss maintenance: a meta-analysis of US studies." *Am. J. Clin. Nutr.* 74 (2001): 579–84.

Behme, M. T., and J. Dupre. "All bran vs corn flakes: plasma glucose and insulin responses in young females." *Am. J. Clin. Nutr.* 50 (1989): 1240-43.

Blatt, A. D., L. S. Roe, and B. J. Rolls, "Hidden vegetables: an effective strategy to reduce energy intake and increase vegetable intake in adults." *Am. J. Clin. Nutr.* 93 (2011): 756–63.

Blom, W. A., et al. "Effect of a high-protein breakfast on the postprandial ghrelin response." *Am. J. Clin. Nutr.* 83 (2006): 211–20.

Chung, K. H., et al. "Study on the obesity and nutrition status of housewives in Seoul and Kyunggi area." *Nutr. Res. Pract.* 5 (2011): 140–94.

Coppinger, T., et al. "Body mass, frequency of eating and breakfast consumption in 9-13-year-olds." *J. Hum. Nutr. Diet.*, 2011 Jun 8, doi:10.1111/j.1365-277X.2011.01184.x.

Davis, L. M., et al. "Efficacy of a meal replacement diet plan compared to a food-based diet plan after a period of weight loss and weight maintenance: a randomized controlled trial." *Nutr. J.* 9 (2010): 11.

de Jong, E., et al. "Behavioural and socio-demographic characteristics of Dutch neighbourhoods with high prevalence of childhood obesity." *Int. J. Pediatr. Obes.* 2011 Jun 27.

Farshchi, H. R., M. A. Taylor, and I. A. Macdonald. "Deleterious effects of omitting breakfast on insulin sensitivity and fasting lipid profiles in healthy lean women." *Am. J. Clin. Nutr.* 81 (2005): 388–96.

Fonda, S. J., A. Jain, and R. A. Vigersky. "A head-to-head comparison of the postprandial effects of 3 meal replacement beverages among people with type 2 diabetes." *Diabetes Educ.* 36 (2010): 793–800.

Gotthelf, L. "Commercial weight loss programs." *Ann. Intern. Med.* 142 (2005): 1023–24; author reply 1024–25.

Hamdy, O., and D. Zwiefelhofer. "Weight management using a meal replacement strategy in type 2 diabetes." *Curr. Diab. Rep.* 10 (2010): 159–64.

Harvey, K., et al. "Eating patterns in patients with spectrum binge-eating disorder." *Int. J. Eat. Disord.* 44 (2011), doi:10.1002/eat.20839.

Hetherington, M. M., and M. F. Regan. "Effects of chewing gum on short-term appetite regulation in moderately restrained eaters." *Appetite*, 2011 Jun 27.

Hill, B. R., M. J. De Souza, and N. I. Williams. "Characterization of the diurnal rhythm of peptide YY and its association with energy balance parameters in normal weight premenopausal women." *Am. J. Physiol. Endocrinol. Metab.,* 2011 May 24.

Holt, S. H., et al. "The effects of high-carbohydrate vs high-fat breakfasts on feelings of fullness and alertness, and subsequent food intake." *Int. J. Food Sci. Nutr.* 50 (1999): 13–28.

Jones, J. M., and J. W. Anderson. "Grain foods and health: a primer for clinicians." *Phys. Sportsmed.* 36 (2008): 18–33.

Kaplan, G. D., and L. T. Stifler. "Very low-calorie diets for obesity." *JAMA* 271 (1994): 24–25.

Kim, J. Y., et al. "Meal replacement with mixed rice is more effective than white rice in weight control, while improving antioxidant enzyme activity in obese women." *Nutr. Res.* 28 (2008): 66–71.

Kral, T. V., et al. "Effects of doubling the portion size of fruit and vegetable side dishes on children's intake at a meal." *Obesity* (Silver Spring) 18 (2010): 521–27.

Leahy, K. E., L. L. Birch, and B. J. Rolls. "Reducing the energy density of an entrée decreases children's energy intake at lunch." *J. Am. Diet Assoc.* 108 (2008): 41–48.

Leahy, K. E., L. L. Birch, and B. J. Rolls. "Reducing the energy density of multiple meals decreases the energy intake of preschool-age children." *Am. J. Clin. Nutr.* 88 (2008): 1459–68.

Levitsky, D. A., and C. Pacanowski. "Losing weight without dieting. Use of commercial foods as meal replacements for lunch produces an extended energy deficit." *Appetite*, 2011 May 11.

Makris A. P., et al. "The individual and combined effects of glycemic index and protein on glycemic response, hunger, and energy intake." *Obesity* (Silver Spring), 2011 Jun 30, doi:10.1038/oby.2011.145.

Marmonier, C., D. Chapelot, and J. Louis-Sylvestre. "Effects of macronutrient content and energy density of snacks consumed in a satiety state on the onset of the next meal." *Appetite* 34 (2000): 161–68.

National Weight Control Registry, http://www.nwcr.ws/Research/default.htm

Osterholt, K. M., L. S. Roe, and B. J. Rolls. "Incorporation of air into a snack food reduces energy intake." *Appetite* 48 (2007): 351–58.

Pombo-Rodrigues, S., W. Calame, and R. Re. "The effects of consuming eggs for lunch on satiety and subsequent food intake." *Int. J. Food Sci. Nutr.,* 2011 Apr 18.

Poole, C. N., et al. "The combined effects of exercise and ingestion of a meal replacement in conjunction with a weight loss supplement on body composition and fitness parameters in college-aged men and women." *J. Strength Cond. Res.* 25 (2011): 51–60.

Purslow, L. R., et al. "Energy intake at breakfast and weight change: prospective study of 6,764 middle-aged men and women." *Am. J. Epidemiol.* 167 (2008): 188–92.

Ratliff, J., et al. "Consuming eggs for breakfast influences plasma glucose and ghrelin, while reducing energy intake during the next 24 hours in adult men." *Nutr. Res.* 30 (2010): 96–103.

Rodríguez-Rodríguez, E., et al. "An adequate calcium intake could help achieve weight loss in overweight/obese women following hypocaloric diets." *Ann. Nutr. Metab.* 57 (2010): 95–102.

Rolls, B. J. "The relationship between dietary energy density and energy intake." *Physiol. Behav.* 97 (2009): 609–15.

Rolls, B. J., A. Drewnowski, and J. H. Ledikwe. "Changing the energy density of the diet as a strategy for weight management." *J. Am. Diet. Assoc.* 105 (2005): S98–103.

Rolls, B. J., et al. "Provision of foods differing in energy density affects long-term weight loss." *Obes. Res.* 13 (2005): 1052–60.

Rolls, B. J., L. S. Roe, and J. S. Meengs. "Portion size can be used strategically to increase vegetable consumption in adults." *Am. J. Clin. Nutr.* 91 (2010): 913–22.

Rolls, B. J., L. S. Roe, and J. S. Meengs. "Reductions in portion size and energy density of foods are additive and lead to sustained decreases in energy intake." *Am. J. Clin. Nutr.* 83 (2006): 11–17.

Sirtori, C. R., et al. "Functional foods for dyslipidaemia and cardiovascular risk prevention." *Nutr. Res. Rev.* 22 (2009): 244–61.

So, H. K., et al. "Breakfast frequency inversely associated with BMI and body fatness in Hong Kong Chinese children aged 9-18 years." *Br. J. Nutr.*, 2011 May 3.

Spill, M. K., et al. "Eating vegetables first: the use of portion size to increase vegetable intake in preschool children." *Am. J. Clin. Nutr.* 91 (2010): 1237–43.

Spill, M. K., et al. "Serving large portions of vegetable soup at the start of a meal affected children's energy and vegetable intake." *Appetite* 57 (2011): 213–19.

Treyzon, L., et al. "A controlled trial of protein enrichment of meal replacements for weight reduction with retention of lean body mass." *Nutr. J.* 7 (2008): 23.

Vander Wal, J. S., et al. "Short-term effect of eggs on satiety in overweight and obese subjects." *J. Am. Coll. Nutr.* 24 (2005): 510–15.

Vander Wal, J. S., et al. "Egg breakfast enhances weight loss." *Int. J. Obes.* (Lond.) 32 (2008): 1545–51.

Chapter 3 Resources

Abete, I., et al. "Obesity and the metabolic syndrome: role of different dietary macronutrient distribution patterns and specific nutritional components on weight loss and maintenance." *Nutr. Rev.* 68 (2010): 214–31.

Appleton, K. M., et al. "Effects of a sweet and a nonsweet lunch on short-term appetite: differences in female high and low consumers of sweet/low-energy beverages." *J. Human Nutr. Diet.* 17 (2004): 425–34.

Barth, S., et al. "Expression of neuropeptide Y, omentin and visfatin in visceral and subcutaneous adipose tissues in humans: relation to endocrine and clinical parameters." *Obes. Facts* (Aug 2010): PMID 20823688.

Beck, B., "Neuropeptide Y in normal eating and in genetic and dietary-induced obesity." *Philos. Trans. R. Soc. Lond. B. Biol. Sci.* 361 (2006): 1159–85.

Blom, W. A., et al. "Effect of a high-protein breakfast on the postprandial ghrelin response." *Am. J. Clin. Nutr.* 83 (2006): 211–20.

Blundell, J. E., and A. J. Hill. "Paradoxical effects of an intense sweetener (aspartame) on appetite." *Lancet* 1 (1986): 1092–93.

Bornet, F. R., et al. "Glycaemic response to foods: impact on satiety and long-term weight regulation." *Appetite* 49 (2007): 535–53.

Chaabo, F., et al. "Nutritional correlates and dynamics of diabetes in the Nile rat (Arvicanthis niloticus): a novel model for diet-induced type 2 diabetes and the metabolic syndrome." *Nutr. Metab.* (Lond.) 7 (2010): 29.

Crespillo, A., et al. "Expression of the cannabinoid system in muscle: effects of a high-fat diet and CB1 receptor blockade." *Biochem. J.* 433 (2010): 175–85.

da S. Benetti, C., et al. "Could preference for palatable foods in neonatally handled rats alter metabolic patterns in adult life?" *Pediatr. Res.* 62 (2007): 405–11.

da S. Benetti, C., et al. "Effects of a chronic exposure to a highly palatable diet and its withdrawal, in adulthood, on cerebral Na+,K+-ATPase and plasma S100B in neonatally handled rats." *Int. J. Dev. Neurosci.* 28 (2010): 153–59.

Davidson, T. L., and S. E. Swithers. "A Pavlovian approach to the problem of obesity." *Int. J. Obes.* 28 (2004): 933–35.

Després, J. P. "The endocannabinoid system: a new target for the regulation of energy balance and metabolism." *Crit. Pathw. Cardiol.* 6 (2007): 46–50.

Di Marzo, V., et al. "Leptin-regulated endocannabinoids are involved in maintaining food intake." *Nature.* 410 (2001): 822–25.

Dulloo, A. G., et al. "Efficacy of a green tea extract rich in catechin polyphenols and caffeine in increasing 24-h energy expenditure and fat oxidation in humans." *Am. J. Clin. Nutr.* 70 (1999): 1040–45.

Francès, F., et al. "The 1258 G>A polymorphism in the neuropeptide Y gene is associated with greater alcohol consumption in a Mediterranean population." *Alcohol* (Mar 2011): PMID 21303710.

Fulton, S. "Appetite and reward." *Front. Neuroendocrinol.* 31 (2010): 85–103.

Gutierrez-Aguilar, R., et al. "Expression of new loci associated with obesity in diet-induced obese rats: from genetics to physiology." *Obesity* (Silver Spring), Jul 2011, doi:10.1038/oby.2011.236.

Guy, E. G., E. Choi, and W. E. Pratt. "Nucleus accumbens dopamine and mu-opioid receptors modulate the reinstatement of food-seeking behavior by food-associated cues." *Behav. Brain Res.* 219 (2011): 265–72.

Hammond, R. A. "Complex systems modeling for obesity research." *Prev. Chronic. Dis.* 6 (2009): A97.

Hanson, E. S., and M. F. Dallman. "Neuropeptide Y (NPY) may integrate responses of hypothalamic feeding systems and the hypothalamo-pituitary-adrenal axis." *J. Neuroendocrinol.* 7 (1995): 273–79.

Henry, C. J., H. J. Lightowler, and C. M. Strik. "Effects of long-term intervention with low- and high-glycaemic-index breakfasts on food intake in children aged 8-11 years." *Br. J. Nutr.* 98 (2007): 636–40.

Holick, M. F., et al. "Evaluation, treatment, and prevention of vitamin D deficiency: an endocrine society clinical practice guideline." *J. Clin. Endocrinol. Metab.* 96 (2011): 1911–30.

Holt, S. H., et al. "The effects of high-carbohydrate vs high-fat breakfasts on feelings of fullness and alertness, and subsequent food intake." *Int. J. Food Sci. Nutr.* 50 (1999): 13–28.

Hursel, R., W. Viechtbauer, and M. S. Westerterp-Plantenga. "The effects of green tea on weight loss and weight maintenance: a meta-analysis." *Int. J. Obes.* (Lond.) 33 (2009): 956–61.

Ilhan, A., et al. "Plasma neuropeptide Y levels differ in distinct diabetic conditions." *Neuropeptides* (Dec 2010): PMID 20832114.

Jakubowicz, D. J., et al. "Effect of diet with high carbohydrate and protein breakfast on weight loss and appetite in obese women with metabolic syndrome." *Endocrine News* 33 (2008): 12.

Johnston, C. S., et al. "Examination of the antiglycemic properties of vinegar in healthy adults." *Ann. Nutr. Metab.* 56 (2010): 74–79.

Kim, E. K., et al. "Fermented kimchi reduces body weight and improves metabolic parameters in overweight and obese patients." *Nutr. Res.* 31 (2011): 436–43.

Kondo, T., et al. "Vinegar intake reduces body weight, body fat mass, and serum triglyceride levels in obese Japanese subjects." *Biosci. Biotechnol. Biochem.* 73 (2009): 1837–43.

Kuo, L. E., et al. "Neuropeptide Y acts directly in the periphery on fat tissue and mediates stress-induced obesity and metabolic syndrome." *Nature Medicine* 13 (2007): 803–11.

Lafrance, V., et al. "Leptin modulates cell morphology and cytokine release in microglia." *Brain Behav. Immun.* 24 (2010): 358–65.

Lee, Y. B., A. Nagai, and S. U. Kim. "Cytokines, chemokines, and cytokine receptors in human microglia." *J. Neurosci. Res.* 69 (2002): 94–103.

Leeman, M., E. Ostman, and I. Björck. "Glycaemic and satiating properties of potato products." *Eur. J. Clin. Nutr.* 62 (2008): 87–95.

Leeman, M., E. Ostman, and I. Björck. "Vinegar dressing and cold storage of potatoes lowers postprandial glycaemic and insulinaemic responses in healthy subjects." *Eur. J. Clin. Nutr.* 59 (2005): 1266–71.

Leibowitz, S. F. "The role of serotonin in eating disorders." *Drugs* 39 (1990): S33–48.

Levy, D. T., et al. "Simulation models of obesity: a review of the literature and implications for research and policy." *Obes. Rev.* 12 (2011), doi:10.1111/j.1467-789X.2010.00804.x.

Liatis, S., et al. "Vinegar reduces postprandial hyperglycaemia in patients with type II diabetes when added to a high, but not to a low, glycaemic index meal." *Eur. J. Clin. Nutr.* 64 (2010): 727–32.

Mozaffarian, D., et al. "Changes in diet and lifestyle and long-term weight gain in women and men." *N. Engl. J. Med.* 364 (2011): 2392–2404.

National Center for Biotechnology Information, U.S. National Library of Medicine website, http://www.ncbi.nlm.nih.gov/gene/4852

Noda, K., et al. "An animal model of spontaneous metabolic syndrome: Nile grass rat." *FASEB J.* 24 (2010): 2443–53.

Ostman, E., et al. "Vinegar supplementation lowers glucose and insulin responses and increases satiety after a bread meal in healthy subjects." *Eur. J. Clin. Nutr.* 59 (2005): 983–88.

Pan, W., et al. "Astrocytes modulate distribution and neuronal signaling of leptin in the hypothalamus of obese A vy mice." *J. Mol. Neurosci.* 43 (2011): 478–84.

Prior, L. J., and J. A. Armitage. "Neonatal overfeeding leads to developmental programming of adult obesity: you are what you ate." *J. Physiol.* 587 (2009): 2419.

Raben, A., et al. "Meals with similar energy densities but rich in protein, fat, carbohydrate, or alcohol have different effects on energy expenditure and substrate metabolism but not on appetite and energy intake." *Am. J. Clin. Nutr.* 77 (2003): 91–100.

Rodrigues, A. L., et al. "Postnatal early overfeeding induces hypothalamic higher SOCS3 expression and lower STAT3 activity in adult rats." *J. Nutr. Biochem.* 22 (2011): 109–17.

Rodrigues, A. L., et al. "Postnatal early overnutrition changes the leptin signaling pathway in the hypothalamic-pituitary-thyroid axis of young and adult rats." *J. Physiol.* 587 (2009): 2647–61.

Sahu, A. "Minireview: A hypothalamic role in energy balance with special emphasis on leptin." *Endocrinology* 145 (2004): 2613–20.

Sclafani, A., K. Touzani, and R. J. Bodnar. "Dopamine and learned food preferences." *Physiol. Behav.* 104 (2011): 64–68.

Skibicka, K. P., et al. "Role of ghrelin in food reward: impact of ghrelin on sucrose self-administration and mesolimbic dopamine and acetylcholine receptor gene expression." *Addict. Biol.*, Feb 2011, doi:10.1111/j.1369-1600.2010.00294.x.

Stellman, S. D., and L. Garfinkel. "Artificial sweetener use and one-year weight change among women." *Preventive Medicine* 15 (1986): 195–202.

Stofkova, A,. et al. "Activation of hypothalamic NPY, AgRP, MC4R, AND IL-6 mRNA levels in young Lewis rats with early-life diet-induced obesity." *Endocr. Regul.* 43 (2009): 99–106.

Sugiyama, S., et al. "Bioavailability of acetate from two vinegar supplements: capsule and drink." *J. Nutr. Sci. Vitaminol.* (Tokyo) 56 (2010): 266–69.

Swithers, S. E., and T. L. Davidson. "A role for sweet taste: calorie predictive relations in energy regulation by rats." *Behav. Neuroscience* 122 (2008): 161–73.

Swithers, S. E., and T. L. Davidson. "Obesity: outwitting the wisdom of the body?" *Curr. Neurol. Neurosci. Rep.* 5 (2005): 159–62.

Swithers, S. E., et al. "General and persistent effects of high-intensity sweeteners on body weight gain and caloric compensation in rats." *Behav. Neuroscience* 123 (2009): 772–80.

Swithers, S. E., et al. "Fat substitutes promote weight gain in rats consuming high-fat diets." *Behav. Neuroscience* 125 (2011): 512–18.

Tapia-González, S., et al. "Activation of microglia in specific hypothalamic nuclei and the cerebellum of adult rats exposed to neonatal overnutrition." *J. Neuroendocrinol.* 23 (2011), doi:10.1111/j.1365-2826.2011.02113.x.

Thaler, J. P., et al. "Hypothalamic inflammation and energy homeostasis: resolving the paradox." *Front Neuroendocrinol.* 31 (2010): 79–84.

Volkow, N. D., G. J. Wang, and R. D. Baler. "Reward, dopamine and the control of food intake: implications for obesity." *Trends Cogn. Sci.* 15 (2011): 37–46.

Wang, J., et al. "Neuropeptide Y in relation to carbohydrate intake, corticosterone and dietary obesity." *Brain Res.* 802 (1998): 75–88.

Wang, G. J., et al. "Brain dopamine and obesity." *The Lancet* 357 (2001): 354–57.

Warren, J. M., C. J. Henry, and V. Simonite. "Low glycemic index breakfasts and reduced food intake in preadolescent children." *Pediatrics* 11 (2003): e414.

Westerterp-Plantenga, M. S. "Green tea catechins, caffeine and body-weight regulation." *Physiol. Behav.* 100 (2010): 42–46.

White, B. D., et al. "Low protein diets increase neuropeptide Y gene expression in the basomedial hypothalamus of rats." *J. Nutr.* 124 (1994): 1152–60.

Young, S. N. "How to increase serotonin in the human brain without drugs." *J. Psychiatry Neurosci.* 32 (2007): 394–99.

Chapter 4 Resources

Abou-Doniaa, M. B., et al. "Splenda alters gut microflora and increases intestinal P-glycoprotein and cytochrome P-450 in male rats." *J. Toxicology Environ. Health* 71 (2008): 1415–29.

Avena, N. M., P. Rada, and B. G. Hoebel. "Evidence for sugar addiction: behavioral and neurochemical effects of intermittent, excessive sugar intake." *Neurosci. Biobehav. Rev.* 32 (2008): 20–39.

Avena, N. M. "Examining the addictive-like properties of binge eating using an animal model of sugar dependence." *Exp. Clin. Psychopharmacol.* 15 (2007): 481–91.

Barth, K. S., et al. "Food cravings and the effects of left prefrontal repetitive transcranial magnetic stimulation using an improved sham condition." *Front. Psychiatry* 2 (2011): 9.

Birch, L. L., and K. K. Davison. "Family environmental factors influencing the developing behavioral controls of food intake and childhood overweight." *Pediatr. Clin. North Am.* 48 (2001): 893–907.

Blum, K., et al. "Reward circuitry dopaminergic activation regulates food and drug craving behavior." *Curr. Pharm. Des.* 17 (2011): 1158–67.

Bruinsma, K., and D. L. Taren. "Chocolate: food or drug?" *J. Am. Diet. Assoc.* 99 (1999): 1249–56.

Corsica, J. A., and B. J. Spring. "Carbohydrate craving: a double-blind, placebo-controlled test of the self-medication hypothesis." *Eat. Behav.* 9 (2008): 447–54.

Harvey, K., E. Kemps, and M. Tiggemann. "The nature of imagery processes underlying food cravings." *Br. J. Health Psychol.* 10 (2005): 49–56.

Hawk, L. W., Jr., et al. "Craving and startle modification during in vivo exposure to food cues." *Appetite* 43 (2004): 285–94.

Hill, A. J. "The psychology of food craving." *Proc. Nutr. Soc.* 66 (2007): 277–85.

Hofmann, W., et al. "As pleasure unfolds. Hedonic responses to tempting food." *Psychol. Sci.* 21 (2010): 1863–70.

Hormes, J. M., and P. Rozin. "Perimenstrual chocolate craving. What happens after menopause?" *Appetite* 53 (2009): 256–9.

Juarascio, A., et al. "The development and validation of the food craving acceptance and action questionnaire (FAAQ)." *Eat. Behav.* 12 (2011): 182–87.

Karhunen, L. J., et al. "Serum leptin, food intake and preferences for sugar and fat in obese women." *Int. J. Obes. Relat. Metab. Disord.* 22 (1998): 819–21.

Kemps, E., et al. "Reduction of food cravings through concurrent visuospatial processing." *Int. J. Eat. Disord.* 36 (2004): 31–40.

Kemps, E., M. Tiggemann, and G. Hart. "Chocolate cravings are susceptible to visuo-spatial interference." *Eat. Behav.* 6 (2005): 101–17.

Kemps, E., and M. Tiggemann. "Attentional bias for craving-related (chocolate) food cues." *Exp. Clin. Psychopharmacol.* 17 (2009): 425–33.

Knäuper, B. "Replacing craving imagery with alternative pleasant imagery reduces craving intensity." *Appetite* 57 (2011): 173–78.

Komatsu, S. "Rice and sushi cravings: a preliminary study of food craving among Japanese females." *Appetite* 50 (2008): 353–58.

Lowe, M. R., and M. L. Butryn. "Hedonic hunger: a new dimension of appetite?" *Physiol. Behav.* 91 (2007): 432–39.

Lundy, R. F., Jr. "Gustatory hedonic value: potential function for forebrain control of brainstem taste processing." *Neurosci. Biobehav. Rev.* 32 (2008): 1601–06.

Macdiarmid, J. I., and M. M. Hetherington. "Mood modulation by food: an exploration of affect and cravings in 'chocolate addicts.'" *Br. J. Clin. Psychol.* 34 (1995): 129–38.

Martin, C. K., et al. "Change in food cravings, food preferences, and appetite during a low-carbohydrate and low-fat diet." *Obesity* (Silver Spring), 2011 Apr 14.

Martin, C. K., et al. "The association between food cravings and consumption of specific foods in a laboratory taste test." *Appetite* 51 (2008): 324–26.

May, J., et al. "Less food for thought. Impact of attentional instructions on intrusive thoughts about snack foods." *Appetite* 55 (2010): 279–87.

Michener, W., et al. "The role of low progesterone and tension as triggers of perimenstrual chocolate and sweets craving: some negative experimental evidence." *Physiol. Behav.* 67 (1999): 417–20.

Ouwehand, C., and E. K. Papies. "Eat it or beat it. The differential effects of food temptations on overweight and normal-weight restrained eaters." *Appetite* 55 (2010): 56–60.

Pelchat, M. L. "Food addiction in humans." *J. Nutr.* 139 (2009): 620–22.

Pelchat, M. L. "Of human bondage: food craving, obsession, compulsion, and addiction." *Physiol. Behav.* 76 (2002): 347–52.

Pickering, C., et al. "Withdrawal from free-choice high-fat high-sugar diet induces craving only in obesity-prone animals." *Psychopharmacology* (Berl) 204 (2009): 431–43.

Polivy, J., J. Coleman, and C. P. Herman. "The effect of deprivation on food cravings and eating behavior in restrained and unrestrained eaters." *Int. J. Eat. Disord.* 38 (2005): 301–09.

Rada, P., N. M. Avena, and B. G. Hoebel. "Daily bingeing on sugar repeatedly releases dopamine in the accumbens shell." *Neuroscience* 134 (2005): 737–44.

Reece, A. S. "Hypothalamic opioid-melanocortin appetitive balance and addictive craving." *Med. Hypotheses* 76 (2011): 132–37.

Rejeski, W. J., et al. "State craving, food availability, and reactivity to preferred snack foods." *Appetite* 54 (2010): 77–83.

Rogers, P. J., and H. J. Smit. "Food craving and food 'addiction': a critical review of the evidence from a biopsychosocial perspective." *Pharmacol. Biochem. Behav.* 66 (2000): 3–14.

Sclafani A., F. Lucas, and K. Ackroff. "The importance of taste and palatability in carbohydrate-induced overeating in rats." *Am. J. Physiol.* 270 (1996): R1197–202.

Sclafani, A. "Psychobiology of food preferences." *Int. J. Obes. Relat. Metab. Disord.* 25 (2001): S13–16.

Siwik, V. P., and J. H. Senf. "Food cravings, ethnicity and other factors related to eating out." *J. Am. Coll. Nutr.* 25 (2006): 382–88.

Tong, J., et al. "Ghrelin enhances olfactory sensitivity and exploratory sniffing in rodents and humans." *J. Neuroscience* 31 (2011), doi:10.1523/JNEUROSCI.5680-10.2011.

Tuomisto, T., et al. "Psychological and physiological characteristics of sweet food 'addiction.'" *Int. J. Eat. Disord.* 25 (1999): 169–75.

Verri, A., et al. "Premenstrual dysphoric disorder and eating disorders." *Cephalalgia* 17 (1997): S25–28.

Weingarten, H. P., and D. Elston. "The phenomenology of food cravings." *Appetite* 15 (1990): 231–46.

Yanovski, S. "Sugar and fat: cravings and aversions." *J. Nutr.* 133 (2003): S835–37.

Yen, J. Y., et al. "The high-sweet-fat food craving among women with premenstrual dysphoric disorder: emotional response, implicit attitude and rewards sensitivity." *Psychoneuroendocrinology* 35 (2010): 1203–12.

Yeomans, M. R., J. E. Blundell, and M. Leshem. "Palatability: response to nutritional need or need-free stimulation of appetite?" *Br. J. Nutr.* 92 (2004): S3–14.

Chapter 5 Resources

Aggarwal, B. B., and K. B. Harikumar. "Potential therapeutic effects of curcumin, the anti-inflammatory agent, against neurodegenerative, cardiovascular, pulmonary, metabolic, autoimmune and neoplastic diseases." *Int. J. Biochem. Cell Biol.* 41 (2009): 40–59.

Aggarwal, B. B., and B. Sung. "Pharmacological basis for the role of curcumin in chronic diseases: an age-old spice with modern targets." *Trends Pharmacol. Sci.* 30 (2009): 85–94.

Ahuja, K. D., et al. "Effects of chili consumption on postprandial glucose, insulin, and energy metabolism." *Am. J. Clin. Nutr.* 84 (2006): 63–69.

Alappat, L., and A. B. Awad. "Curcumin and obesity: evidence and mechanisms." *Nutr. Rev.* 68 (2010), doi:10.1111/j.1753-4887.2010.00341.x.

Alemzadeh, R., et al. "Hypovitaminosis D in obese children and adolescents: relationship with adiposity, insulin sensitivity, ethnicity, and season." *Metabolism* 57 (2008): 183–91.

Anne Moorhead, S., et al. "The effects of the fibre content and physical structure of carrots on satiety and subsequent intakes when eaten as part of a mixed meal." *Br. J. Nutr.* 96 (2006): 587–95.

Barry, J. A., P. Bouloux, and P. J. Hardiman. "The impact of eating behavior on psychological symptoms typical of reactive hypoglycemia." Appetite 57 (2011): 73–76.

Barth, R. J. "Insulin resistance, obesity and the metabolic syndrome." *S. D. Med.* Spec No. (2011): 22–27.

Bastard, J. P., et al. "Recent advances in the relationship between obesity, inflammation, and insulin resistance." *Eur. Cytokine Netw.* 17 (2006): 4–12.

Belza, A., E. Frandsen, and J. Kondrup. "Body fat loss achieved by stimulation of thermogenesis by a combination of bioactive food ingredients: a placebo-controlled, double-blind 8-week intervention in obese subjects." *Int. J. Obes.* (Lond.) 31 (2007): 121–30.

Belza, A., and A. B. Jessen. "Bioactive food stimulants of sympathetic activity: effect on 24-h energy expenditure and fat oxidation." *Eur. J. Clin. Nutr.* 59 (2005): 733–41.

Bodinham, C. L., et al. "Short-term effects of whole-grain wheat on appetite and food intake in healthy adults: a pilot study." *Br. J. Nutr.* 106 (2011): 327–30.

Brun, J. F., et al. "Evaluation of a standardized hyperglucidic breakfast test in postprandial reactive hypoglycaemia." *Diabetologia* 38 (1995): 494–501.

Brun, J. F., C. Fedou, and J. Mercier. "Postprandial reactive hypoglycemia." *Diabetes Metab.* 26 (2000): 337–51.

Caldas, A. D., et al. "Relationship between insulin and hypogonadism in men with metabolic syndrome." *Arq. Bras. Endocrinol. Metabol.* 53 (2009): 1005–11.

Chartoumpekis, D. V., et al. "Brown adipose tissue responds to cold and adrenergic stimulation by induction of FGF21." *Mol. Med.*, Feb 2011, doi:10.2119/molmed.2011.00075.

Chen, N., et al. "Green tea, black tea, and epigallocatechin modify body composition, improve glucose tolerance, and differentially alter metabolic gene expression in rats fed a high-fat diet." *Nutr. Res.* 29 (2009): 784–93.

Chi, Q. S., and D. H. Wang. "Thermal physiology and energetics in male desert hamsters (Phodopus roborovskii) during cold acclimation." *J. Comp. Physiol. B.* 181 (2011): 91–103.

Després, J. P., et al. "Abdominal obesity and the metabolic syndrome: contribution to global cardiometabolic risk." *Arterioscler. Thromb, Vasc. Biol.* 28 (2008): 1039–49.

Diepvens, K., et al. "Obesity and thermogenesis related to the consumption of caffeine, ephedrine, capsaicin, and green tea." *Am. J. Physiol. Regul. Integr. Comp. Physiol.* 292 (2007): R77–85.

Dittrich, R., et al. "Association of thyroid-stimulating hormone with insulin resistance and androgen parameters in women with PCOS." *Reprod. Biomed. Online* 19 (2009): 319–25.

Dixit, A. A., et al. "Incorporation of whole, ancient grains into a modern Asian Indian diet to reduce the burden of chronic disease." *Nutr. Rev.* 69 (2011), doi:10.1111/j.1753-4887.2011.00411.x.

Duvnjak, L., and M. Duvnjak. "The metabolic syndrome—an ongoing story." *J. Physiol. Pharmacol.* (Dec 2009): S19–24.

Fain, J. N. "Release of interleukins and other inflammatory cytokines by human adipose tissue is enhanced in obesity and primarily due to the nonfat cells." *Vitam. Horm.* 74 (2006): 443–77.

Galgani, J. E., and E. Ravussin. "Effect of dihydrocapsiate on resting metabolic rate in humans." *Am. J. Clin. Nutr.* 92 (2010): 1089–93.

Goudas, V. T., and D. A. Dumesic. "Polycystic ovary syndrome." *Endocrinol Metab. Clin. North Am.* 26 (1997): 893–912.

Griggio, M. A. "Thermogenic mechanisms in cold-acclimated animals." *Braz. J. Med. Biol. Res.* 21 (1988): 171–76.

Gruenwald, J., J. Freder, and N. Armbruester. "Cinnamon and health." *Crit. Rev. Food Sci. Nutr.* 50 (2010): 822–34.

Guay, A. T. "The emerging link between hypogonadism and metabolic syndrome." *J. Androl.* 30 (2009): 370–76.

Harach, T., et al. "Rosemary (Rosmarinus officinalis L.) leaf extract limits weight gain and liver steatosis in mice fed a high-fat diet." *Planta Med.* 76 (2010): 566–71.

Harada, K., et al. "Resistance to high-fat diet-induced obesity and altered expression of adipose-specific genes in HSL-deficient mice." *Am. J. Physiol. Endocrinol. Metab.* 285 (2003): E1182–95.

Hlebowicz, J., et al. "Effect of commercial breakfast fibre cereals compared with corn flakes on postprandial blood glucose, gastric emptying and satiety in healthy subjects: a randomized blinded crossover trial." *Nutr. J.* 6 (2007): 22.

Hlebowicz, J., et al. "Effect of muesli with 4 g oat beta-glucan on postprandial blood glucose, gastric emptying and satiety in healthy subjects: a randomized crossover trial." *J. Am. Coll. Nutr.* 27 (2008): 470–75.

Hlebowicz, J., et al. "The botanical integrity of wheat products influences the gastric distention and satiety in healthy subjects." *Nutr. J.* 7 (2008): 12.

Hofeldt, F. D. "Reactive hypoglycemia." *Endocrinol. Metab. Clin. North Am.* 18 (1989): 185–201.

Hondares, E. "Thermogenic activation induces FGF21 expression and release in brown adipose tissue." *J. Biol. Chem.* 286 (2011): 12983–90.

Hursel, R., and M. S. Westerterp-Plantenga. "Thermogenic ingredients and body weight regulation." *Int. J. Obes.* (Lond.) 34 (2010): 659–69.

Ibarra, A., et al. "Carnosic acid-rich rosemary (Rosmarinus officinalis L.) leaf extract limits weight gain and improves cholesterol levels and glycaemia in mice on a high-fat diet." *Br. J. Nutr.* 17 (2011): 1–8.

Islam, M. S., and H. Choi. "Antidiabetic effect of Korean traditional Baechu (Chinese cabbage) kimchi in a type 2 diabetes model of rats." *J. Med. Food* 12 (2009): 292–97.

Islam, M. S., and H. Choi. "Comparative effects of dietary ginger (Zingiber officinale) and garlic (Allium sativum) investigated in a type 2 diabetes model of rats." *J. Med. Food* 11 (2008): 152–59.

Jerzsa-Latta, M., M. Krondl, and P. Coleman. "Use and perceived attributes of cruciferous vegetables in terms of genetically-mediated taste sensitivity." *Appetite* 15 (1990): 127–34.

Jones, T. H. "Effects of testosterone on Type 2 diabetes and components of the metabolic syndrome." *J. Diabetes* 2 (2010), doi:10.1111/j.1753-0407.2010.00085.x.

Kirkham, S., et al. "The potential of cinnamon to reduce blood glucose levels in patients with type 2 diabetes and insulin resistance." *Diabetes Obes. Metab.* 11 (2009): 1100–13.

Kirsty Forsythe, L., et al. "Effect of adiposity on vitamin D status and the 25-hydroxycholecalciferol response to supplementation in healthy young and older Irish adults." *Br. J. Nutr.* 28 (2011): 1–9.

Kral, T. V. "Effects on hunger and satiety, perceived portion size and pleasantness of taste of varying the portion size of foods: a brief review of selected studies." *Appetite* 46 (2006): 103–05.

Kristensen, M., et al. "Wholegrain vs. refined wheat bread and pasta. Effect on postprandial glycemia, appetite, and subsequent ad libitum energy intake in young healthy adults." *Appetite* 54 (2010): 163–69.

Landis, A. M., K. P. Parker, and S. B. Dunbar. "Sleep, hunger, satiety, food cravings, and caloric intake in adolescents." *J. Nurs. Scholarsh.* 41 (2009): 115–23.

LaZovic, G., et al. "Influence of adiposity on leptin, LH and androgen levels in lean, overweight and obese PCOS patients." *Int. J. Fertil. Women's Med.* 52 (2007): 82–88.

Madkor, H. R., S. W. Mansour, and G. Ramadan. "Modulatory effects of garlic, ginger, turmeric and their mixture on hyperglycaemia, dyslipidaemia and oxidative stress in streptozotocin-nicotinamide diabetic rats." *Br. J. Nutr.* 105 (2011): 1210–17.

Makhsida, N., et al. "Hypogonadism and metabolic syndrome: implications for testosterone therapy." *J. Urol.* 174 (2005): 827–34.

Marinangeli, C. P., and P. J. Jones. "Functional food ingredients as adjunctive therapies to pharmacotherapy for treating disorders of metabolic syndrome." *Ann. Med.* 42 (2010): 317–33.

Marinangeli, C. P., and P. J. Jones. "Plant sterols, marine-derived omega-3 fatty acids and other functional ingredients: a new frontier for treating hyperlipidemia." *Nutr. Metab.* (Lond.) 7 (2010): 76.

Marsh, K. A., et al. "Effect of a low glycemic index compared with a conventional healthy diet on polycystic ovary syndrome." *Am. J. Clin. Nutr.* 92 (2010): 83–92.

Moriarty-Kelsey, M., et al. "Testosterone, obesity and insulin resistance in young males: evidence for an association between gonadal dysfunction and insulin resistance during puberty." *J. Pediatr. Endocrinol. Metab.* 23 (2010): 1281–87.

Mueller, M., et al. "Oregano: a source for peroxisome proliferator-activated receptor gamma antagonists." *J. Agric. Food Chem.* 56 (2008): 11621–30.

Ngo, D. T., et al. "Determinants of insulin responsiveness in young women: impact of polycystic ovarian syndrome, nitric oxide, and vitamin D." *Nitric Oxide*, 2011 Jun 30.

Ottenhof, M. A., S. E. Hill, and I. A. Farhat. "Comparative study of the retrogradation of intermediate water content waxy maize, wheat, and potato starches." *J. Agric. Food Chem.* 53 (2005): 631–38.

Pacifico, L., et al. "Low 25(OH)D3 levels are associated with total adiposity, metabolic syndrome, and hypertension in Caucasian children and adolescents." *Eur. J. Endocrinol.*, 2011 Jul 13.

Pittas, A. G., et al. "The role of vitamin D and calcium in type 2 diabetes. A systematic review and meta-analysis." *J. Clin. Endocrinol. Metab.* 92 (2007): 2017–29.

Ros Pérez, M., and G. Medina-Gómez. "Obesity, adipogenesis and insulin resistance." *Endocrinol. Nutr.*, 2011 Jul 19.

Roussel, A. M., et al. "Antioxidant effects of a cinnamon extract in people with impaired fasting glucose that are overweight or obese." *Am. Coll. Nutr.* 28 (2009): 16–21.

Ruf, T., and B. Grafl. "Maximum rates of sustained metabolic rate in cold-exposed Djungarian hamsters (Phodopus sungorus): the second wind." *J. Comp. Physiol. B.* 180 (2010): 1089–98.

Sadiq Butt, M., et al. "Oat: unique among the cereals." *Eur. J. Nutr.* 47 (2008): 68–79.

Sengupta, A., and M. Ghosh. "Hypolipidemic effect of mustard oil enriched with medium chain fatty acid and polyunsaturated fatty acid." *Nutrition*, 2011 May 27.

Setji, T. L., and A. J. Brown. "Comprehensive clinical management of polycystic ovary syndrome." *Minerva Med.* 98 (2007): 175–89.

Shah, S. S., et al. "Effect of piperine in the regulation of obesity-induced dyslipidemia in high-fat diet rats." *Indian J. Pharmacol.* 43 (2011): 296–99.

Silfen, M. E., et al. "Early endocrine, metabolic, and sonographic characteristics of polycystic ovary syndrome (PCOS): comparison between nonobese and obese adolescents." *J. Clin. Endocrinol. Metab.* 88 (2003): 4682–88.

Spritzer, P. M., et al. "Leptin concentrations in hirsute women with polycystic ovary syndrome or idiopathic hirsutism: influence on LH and relationship with hormonal, metabolic, and anthropometric measurements." *Hum. Reprod.* 16 (2001): 1340–46.

Su, Q., et al. "Identification and quantitation of major carotenoids in selected components of the Mediterranean diet: green leafy vegetables, figs and olive oil." *Eur. J. Clin. Nutr.* 56 (2002): 1149–54.

Traish, A. M., et al. "The dark side of testosterone deficiency: I. Metabolic syndrome and erectile dysfunction." *J. Androl.* 30 (2009): 10–22.

Trayhurn, P., and I. S. Wood. "Adipokines: inflammation and the pleiotropic role of white adipose tissue." *Br. J. Nutr.* 92 (2004): 347–55.

Tremblay, A., and J. A. Gilbert. "Milk products, insulin resistance syndrome and type 2 diabetes." *J. Am. Coll. Nutr.* 28 (2009): S91–102.

van Meijl, L. E., and R. P. Mensink. "Effects of low-fat dairy consumption on markers of low-grade systemic inflammation and endothelial function in overweight and obese subjects: an intervention study." *Br. J. Nutr.* 104 (2010): 1523–27.

Vega-Gálvez, A., et al. "Nutrition facts and functional potential of quinoa (Chenopodium quinoa willd.), an ancient Andean grain: a review." *J. Sci. Food Agric.* 90 (2010): 2541–47.

Vijayakumar, R. S., D. Surya, and N. Nalini. "Antioxidant efficacy of black pepper (Piper nigrum L.) and piperine in rats with high fat diet induced oxidative stress." *Redox. Rep.* 9 (2004): 105–10.

Welch, R. W. "Can dietary oats promote health?" *Br. J. Biomed. Sci.* 51 (1994): 260–70.

Wennersberg, M. H., et al. "Dairy products and metabolic effects in overweight men and women: results from a 6-mo intervention study." *Am. J. Clin. Nutr.* 90 (2009): 960–68.

Westerterp-Plantenga, M., et al. "Metabolic effects of spices, teas, and caffeine." *Physiol. Behav.* 89 (2006): 85–91.

Wilkinson, L. L., and J. M. Brunstrom. "Conditioning 'fullness expectations' in a novel dessert." *Appetite* 52 (2009): 780–83.

Wu, H., et al. "Lifestyle counseling and supplementation with flaxseed or walnuts influence the management of metabolic syndrome." *J. Nutr.* 140 (2010): 1937–42.

Yamamoto, M., et al. "Anti-obesity effects of lipase inhibitor CT-II, an extract from edible herbs, Nomame Herba, on rats fed a high-fat diet." *Int. J. Obes. Relat. Metab. Disord.* 24 (2000): 758–64.

Yucel, A., V. Noyan, and N. Sagsoz. "The association of serum androgens and insulin resistance with fat distribution in polycystic ovary syndrome." *Eur. J. Obstet. Gynecol. Reprod. Biol.* 126 (2006): 81–86.

Chapter 6 Resources

Anderson, J. W., et. al. "Health benefits of dietary fiber." *Nutr. Rev.* 67 (2009): 188–205.

Araya, H., et al. "Short-term satiety in preschool children: a comparison between high protein meal and a high complex carbohydrate meal." *Int. J. Food Sci. Nutr.* 51 (2000): 119–24.

Beck, E. J., et al. "Oat beta-glucan supplementation does not enhance the effectiveness of an energy-restricted diet in overweight women." *Br. J. Nutr.* 103 (2010): 1212–22.

Bell, E. A., et al. "Energy density of foods affects energy intake in normal-weight women." *Am. J. Clin. Nutr.* 67 (1998): 412–20.

Bell, E. A., et al. "Sensory-specific satiety is affected more by volume than by energy content of a liquid food." *Physiol. Behav.* 78 (2003): 593–600.

Birketvedt, G. S. "Long-term effect of fibre supplement and reduced energy intake on body weight and blood lipids in overweight subjects." *Acta. Medica.* 43 (2000): 129–32.

Blom, W. A., et al. "Effect of a high-protein breakfast on the postprandial ghrelin response." *Am. J. Clin. Nutr.* 83 (2006): 211–20.

Blundell, J. E., and J. I. MacDiarmid. "Fat as a risk factor for overconsumption: satiation, satiety, and patterns of eating." *J. Am. Diet. Assoc.* 97 (1997): S63–69.

Cheskin, L. J. "Lack of energy compensation over 4 days when white button mushrooms are substituted for beef." *Appetite* 51 (2008): 50–57.

Crum, A. J., et al. "Mind over milkshakes: mindsets, not just nutrients, determine ghrelin response." *Health Psychol.*, 2011 May 16.

Dickson, S. L., et al. "The role of the central ghrelin system in reward from food and chemical drugs." *Mol. Cell. Endocrinol.* 340 (2011): 80–87.

Disse, E., et al. "Systemic ghrelin and reward: effect of cholinergic blockade." *Physiol. Behav.* 102 (2011): 481–84.

Green, S. M., et al. "Effect of fat- and sucrose-containing foods on the size of eating episodes and energy intake in lean males: potential for causing overconsumption," *Eur. J. Clin. Nutr.* 48 (1994): 547–55.

Heini, A. F., et al. "Effect of hydrolyzed guar fiber on fasting and postprandial satiety and satiety hormones: a double-blind, placebo-controlled trial during controlled weight loss." *Int. J. Obes. Relat. Metab. Disord.* 22 (1998): 906–09.

Hellström, P. M., and E. Näslund. "Interactions between gastric emptying and satiety, with special reference to glucagon-like peptide-1." *Physiol. Behav.* 74 (2001): 735–41.

Hlebowicz, J., et al. "Effects of 1 and 3 g cinnamon on gastric emptying, satiety, and postprandial blood glucose, insulin, glucose-dependent insulinotropic polypeptide, glucagon-like peptide 1, and ghrelin concentrations in healthy subjects." *Am. J. Clin. Nutr.* 89 (2009): 815–21.

Holt, S. H., et al. "A satiety index of common foods." *Eur. J. Clin. Nutr.* (Sept 1995): 675–90.

Holt, S. A., et al. "The effects of equal-energy portions of different breads on blood glucose levels, feelings of fullness and subsequent food intake." *J. Amer. Diet. Assoc.* 101 (2001): 767–73.

Howarth, N. C. "Dietary fiber and weight regulation." *Nutr. Rev.* 59 (2001): 129–39.

Howarth, N. C. "Fermentable and nonfermentable fiber supplements did not alter hunger, satiety or body weight in a pilot study of men and women consuming self-selected diets." *J. Nutr.* 133 (2003): 3141–44.

Li, J., et al. "Improvement in chewing activity reduces energy intake in one meal and modulates plasma gut hormone concentrations in obese and lean young Chinese men." *Am. J. Clin. Nutr.* 94 (2011): 709–16.

Marmonier, C., et al. "Effects of macronutrient content and energy density of snacks consumed in a satiety state on the onset of the next meal." *Appetite* 34 (2000): 161–68.

Mattes, R. D., et al. "Beverage viscosity is inversely related to postprandial hunger in humans." *Physiol. Behav.* 74 (2001): 551–57.

Nachtigal, M. C. "Dietary supplements and weight control in a middle-age population." *J. Altern. Complement Med.* 11 (2005): 909–15.

Naleida, A. M., et al. "Ghrelin induces feeding in the mesolimbic reward pathway between the ventral tegmental area and the nucleus accumbens." *Peptides* 26 (2005): 2274–79.

Nieman, D. C., et al. "Chia seed does not promote weight loss or alter disease risk factors in overweight adults." *Nutr. Res.* 29 (2009): 414–18.

Rolls, B. J., et al. "Portion size of food affects energy intake in normal-weight and overweight men and women." *Am. J. Clin. Nutr.* 76 (2002): 1207–13.

Rolls, B. J., et al. "Volume of food consumed affects satiety in men." *Am. J. Clin. Nutr.* 67 (1998): 1170–77.

Rolls, B., et al. "Salad and satiety: eEnergy density and portion size of a first-course salad affect energy intake at lunch." *J. Am. Diet. Assoc.* 107 (2004): 1570–76.

Rolls, B., et al. "Water incorporated into a food but not served with a food decreases energy intake in lean women." *Am. J. Clin. Nutr.* 70 (1999): 448–55.

Salas-Salvadó, J., et al. "Effect of two doses of a mixture of soluble fibres on body weight and metabolic variables in overweight or obese patients: a randomised trial." *Br. J. Nutr.* 99 (2008): 1380–87.

Whybrow, S. "Effects of added fruits and vegetables on dietary intakes and body weight in Scottish adults." *Br. J. Nutr.* 95 (2006): 496–503.

Wood, R. J. "Effects of a carbohydrate-restricted diet with and without supplemental soluble fiber on plasma low-density lipoprotein cholesterol and other clinical markers of cardiovascular risk." *Metabolism* 56 (2007): 58–67.

Chapter 7 Resources

Anderson, B., et al. "Fast-food consumption and obesity among Michigan adults." *Prev. Chronic. Dis.* 8 (2011): A71.

Babaei, A., et al. "Restricted leptin antagonism as a therapeutic approach to treatment of autoimmune diseases." *Hormones* (Athens) 10 (2011): 16–26.

Berthoud, H. R. "Interactions between the 'cognitive' and 'metabolic' brain in the control of food intake." *Physiol. Behav.* 91 (2007): 486–98.

Chakravarthy, M. V., and F. W. Booth. "Eating, exercise, and 'thrifty' genotypes: connecting the dots toward an evolutionary understanding of modern chronic diseases." *J. Appl. Physiol.* 96 (2004): 3–10.

Cornier, M. A. "Is your brain to blame for weight regain?" *Physiol. Behav.,* 2011 Apr 9.

Dalmas, E., et al. "Defining macrophage phenotype and function in adipose tissue." *Trends Immunol.,* 2011 May 25.

Egecioglu, E., et al. "Hedonic and incentive signals for body weight control." *Rev. Endocr. Metab. Disord.,* 2011 Feb 22.

Enriori, P. J., et al. "Diet-induced obesity causes severe but reversible leptin resistance in arcuate melanocortin neurons." *Cell. Metab.* 5 (2007): 181–94.

Espinola-Klein, C., et al. "Inflammatory markers and cardiovascular risk in the metabolic syndrome." *Front. Biosci.* 16 (2011): 1663–74.

Exner, C., et al. "Leptin suppresses semi-starvation induced hyperactivity in rats: implications for anorexia nervosa." *Mol. Psychiatry* 5 (2000): 476–81.

Faggioni, R., et al. "Reduced leptin levels in starvation increase susceptibility to endotoxic shock." *Am. J. Pathol.* 156 (2000): 1781–87.

Fehm, H. L., et al. "The selfish brain: competition for energy resources." *Prog. Brain Res.* 153 (2006): 129–40.

Fernández-Sánchez, A., et al. "Inflammation, oxidative stress, and obesity." *Int. J. Mol. Sci.* 12 (2011): 3117–32.

Furet, J. P., et al. "Differential adaptation of human gut microbiota to bariatric surgery-induced weight loss: links with metabolic and low-grade inflammation markers." *Diabetes* 59 (2010): 3049–57.

Healy, L., et al. "Metabolic syndrome and leptin are associated with adverse Pathological features in male colorectal cancer patients." *Colorectal Dis.* (Jan 2011), doi:10.1111/j.1463-1318.2011.02562.x.

Heikens, M. J., et al. "Core body temperature in obesity." *Am. J. Clin. Nutr.* 93 (2011): 963–67.

Howard, J. .K., et al. "Leptin protects mice from starvation-induced lymphoid atrophy and increases thymic cellularity in ob/ob mice." *J. Clin. Invest.* 104 (1999): 1051–59.

Howard, P. H., et al. "Proximity of food retailers to schools and rates of overweight ninth grade students: an ecological study in California." *BMC Public Health.* 11 (2011): 68.

Huang, X. F., et al. "Role of fat amount and type in ameliorating diet-induced obesity: insights at the level of hypothalamic arcuate nucleus leptin receptor, neuropeptide Y and pro-opiomelanocortin mRNA expression." *Diabetes Obes. Metab.* 6 (2004): 35–44.

Ide, J., et al. "Macrophage-conditioned medium inhibits the activation of cyclin-dependent kinase 2 by adipogenic inducers in 3T3-L1 preadipocytes." *J. Cell. Physiol.* 226 (2011), doi:10.1002/jcp.22566.

Jeon, J. Y., et al. "Leptin response to short-term fasting in sympathectomized men: role of the SNS." *Am. J. Physiol., Endo.* 284 (2003): E634–40.

Jéquier, E. "Leptin signaling, adiposity, and energy balance." *Ann. NY Acad. Sci.* 967 (2002): 379–88.

Kawanishi, N., et al. "Exercise training inhibits inflammation in adipose tissue via both suppression of macrophage infiltration and acceleration of phenotypic switching from M1 to M2 macrophages in high-fat-diet-induced obese mice." *Exerc. Immunol. Rev.* 16 (2010): 105–18.

Klein, S., et al. "Leptin production during early starvation in lean and obese women." *Am. J. Physiol., Endo.* 278 (2000): E280–84.

Lenard, N. R., and H. R. Berthoud. "Central and peripheral regulation of food intake and physical activity: pathways and genes." *Obesity* (Silver Spring) 16 (2008): S11–22.

Makoundou, V., et al. "Do obese patients after weight loss become metabolically normal?" *Obes. Facts* 4 (2011): 218–21.

Mollica, M. P. "From chronic overfeeding to hepatic injury: role of endoplasmic reticulum stress and inflammation." *Nutr. Metab. Cardiovasc. Dis.* 21 (2011): 222–30.

Pandit, R., et al. "Neurobiology of overeating and obesity: the role of melanocortins and beyond." *Eur. J. Pharmacol.* 660 (2011): 28–42.

Park, J., and P. E. Scherer. "Leptin and cancer: from cancer stem cells to metastasis." *Endocr. Relat. Cancer*, 2011 Jun 16.

Peters, A., et al. "Causes of obesity: looking beyond the hypothalamus." *Prog. Neurobiol.* 81 (2007): 61–88.

Peters A., et al. "The selfish brain: competition for energy resources." *Neurosci. Biobehav. Rev.* 28 (2004): 143–80.

Salawu, A. A., et al. "Effect of the juice of lime (Citrus aurantifolia) on estrous cycle and ovulation of Sprague-Dawley rats." *Endocr. Pract.* 16 (2010): 561–65.

So, M., et al. "Analysis of time-dependent adaptations in whole-body energy balance in obesity induced by high-fat diet in rats." *Lipids Health Dis.* 10 (2011): 99.

Surmi, B. K., and A. H. Hasty. "Macrophage infiltration into adipose tissue: initiation, propagation and remodeling." *Future Lipidol.* 3 (2008): 545–56.

Tanaka, M., et al. "Role of central leptin signaling in the starvation-induced alteration of B-cell development." *J. Neurosci.* 31 (2011): 8373–80.

van Dijk, G. "The role of leptin in the regulation of energy balance and adiposity." *J. Neuroendocrinol.* 13 (2001): 913–21.

Wang, H., et al. "Effects of dietary fat types on body fatness, leptin, and ARC leptin receptor, NPY, and AgRP mRNA expression." *Am. J. Physiol. Endocrinol. Metab.* 282 (2002): E1352–59.

Wauman, J., and J. Tavernier. "Leptin receptor signaling: pathways to leptin resistance." *Front Biosci.* 17 (2011): 2771–93.

Wright, S. M., and L. J. Aronne. "Obesity in 2010: the future of obesity medicine: where do we go from here?" *Nat. Rev. Endocrinol.* 7 (2011): 69–70.

Yu, Y., et al. "Obese reversal by a chronic energy restricted diet leaves an increased Arc NPY/AgRP, but no alteration in POMC/CART, mRNA expression in diet-induced obese mice." *Behav. Brain Res.* 205 (2009): 50–56.

Zheng, H., et al. "Appetite control and energy balance regulation in the modern world: reward-driven brain overrides repletion signals." *Int. J. Obes.* (Lond). 33 (2009): S8–13.

Zupancic, M. L., and A. Mahajan. "Leptin as a neuroactive agent." *Psychosom. Med.* 73 (2011): 407–14.

Chapter 8 Resources

Andrés, C. "131I activity in urine to the sewer system due to thyroidal treatments." *Health Phys.* 101 (2011): S110–15.

Arsenescu, V., et al. "Polychlorinated biphenyl-77 induces adipocyte differentiation and proinflammatory adipokines and promotes obesity and atherosclerosis." *Environ. Health Perspect.* 116 (2008): 761–68.

Baer, D. J., et al. "Whey protein but not soy protein supplementation alters body weight and composition in free-living overweight and obese adults." *J. Nutr.*, 2011 Jun 15.

Charlier, C., C. Desaive, and G. Plomteux. "Human exposure to endocrine disrupters: consequences of gastroplasty on plasma concentration of toxic pollutants." *Int. J. Obes. Relat. Metab. Disord.* 26 (2002): 1465–68.

Crawford, B. A., et al. "Iodine toxicity from soy milk and seaweed ingestion is associated with serious thyroid dysfunction." *Med. J. Aust.* 193 (2010): 413–15.

Desvergne, B., J. N. Feige, and C. Casals-Casas. "PPAR-mediated activity of phthalates: a link to the obesity epidemic?" *Mol. Cell Endocrinol.* 304 (2009): 43–48.

Diamanti-Kandarakis, E., et al. "Endocrine-disrupting chemicals: an Endocrine Society scientific statement." *Endocr. Rev.* 30 (2009): 293–342.

Dirinck, E., et al. "Obesity and persistent organic pollutants: possible obesogenic effect of organochlorine pesticides and polychlorinated biphenyls." *Obesity* (Silver Spring) 19 (2011): 709–14.

Doerge, D. R., and H. C. Chang. "Inactivation of thyroid peroxidase by soy isoflavones, in vitro and in vivo." *J. Chromatogr. B. Analyt. Technol. Biomed. Life Sci.* 777 (2002): 269–79.

Doerge, D. R., and D. M. Sheehan. "Goitrogenic and estrogenic activity of soy isoflavones." *Environ. Health Perspect.* 110 (2002): S349–53.

Duhigg, C. "Debating how much weed killer is safe in your water glass." *New York Times*, August 22, 2009.

Environmental Working Group, www.ewg.org/foodnews

Grün, F. "Obesogens." *Curr. Opin. Endocrinol. Diabetes Obes.* 17 (2010): 453–59.

Grün, F., and B. Blumberg. "Endocrine disrupters as obesogens." *Mol. Cell Endocrinol.* 304 (2009): 19–29.

Grün, F., and B. Blumberg. "Environmental obesogens: organotins and endocrine disruption via nuclear receptor signaling." *Endocrinology* 147 (2006): S50–55.

He, K., et al. "Consumption of monosodium glutamate in relation to incidence of overweight in Chinese adults: China Health and Nutrition Survey (CHNS)." *Am. J. Clin. Nutr.* 93 (2011): 1328–36.

Hermansen, K., et al. "Beneficial effects of a soy-based dietary supplement on lipid levels and cardiovascular risk markers in type 2 diabetic subjects." *Diabetes Care* 24 (2001): 228–33.

Hotchkiss, A. K., et al. "Fifteen years after 'Wingspread'—environmental endocrine disrupters and human and wildlife health: where we are today and where we need to go." *Toxicol. Sci.* 105 (2008): 235–59.

Howe, C. M., et al. "Toxicity of glyphosate-based pesticides to four North American frog species." *Environ. Toxicol. Chem.* 23 (2004): 1928–38.

Janesick, A., and B. Blumberg. "Endocrine disrupting chemicals and the developmental programming of adipogenesis and obesity." *Birth Defects Res. C. Embryo Today* 93 (2011), doi:10.1002/bdrc.20197.

Janesick, A., and B. Blumberg. "Minireview: PPARγ as the target of obesogens." *J. Steroid Biochem. Mol. Biol.*, 2011 Jan 18.

Jayagopal, V., et al. "Beneficial effects of soy phytoestrogen intake in postmenopausal women with type 2 diabetes." *Diabetes Care* 25 (2002): 1709–14.

Jobst, K. A. "You are what you eat: stress, survival anxiety, the environment, and chemical obesogens." *J. Altern. Complement. Med.* 8 (2002): 101–02.

Karmaus, W., et al. "Maternal levels of dichlorodiphenyl-dichloroethylene (DDE) may increase weight and body mass index in adult female offspring." *Occup. Environ. Med.* 66 (2009): 143–49.

Kim, M. H., et al. "Genistein and daidzein repress adipogenic differentiation of human adipose tissue-derived mesenchymal stem cells via Wnt/β-catenin signalling or lipolysis." *Cell Prolif.* 43 (2010), doi:10.1111/j.1365-2184.2010.00709.x.

Kirchner, S., et al. "Prenatal exposure to the environmental obesogen tributyltin predisposes multipotent stem cells to become adipocytes." *Mol. Endocrinol.* 24 (2010): 526–39.

Lee, D. H., et al. "Polychlorinated biphenyls and organochlorine pesticides in plasma predict development of type 2 diabetes in the elderly: the Prospective Investigation of the Vasculature in Uppsala Seniors (PIVUS) study." *Diabetes Care*, 2011 Jun 23.

Leung, A. M. "Iodine status and thyroid function of Boston-area vegetarians and vegans." *J. Clin. Endocrinol. Metab.*, 2011 May 25.

Li, X., J. Ycaza, and B. Blumberg. "The environmental obesogen tributyltin chloride acts via peroxisome proliferator activated receptor gamma to induce adipogenesis in murine 3T3-L1 preadipocytes." *J. Steroid Biochem. Mol. Biol.*, 2011 Mar 21.

Martin, A. "Chemical suspected in cancer is in baby products," *New York Times*, May 17, 2011.

McMillan, M., E. A. Spinks, and G. R. Fenwick. "Preliminary observations on the effect of dietary brussels sprouts on thyroid function." *Hum. Toxicol.* 5 (1986): 15–19.

Meador, J. P., et al. "Tributyltin and the obesogen metabolic syndrome in a salmonid." *Environ. Res.* 111 (2011): 50–56.

Naaz, A., et al. "The soy isoflavone genistein decreases adipose deposition in mice." *Endocrinology* 144 (2003): 3315–20.

Penza, M., et al. "Genistein affects adipose tissue deposition in a dose-dependent and gender-specific manner." *Endocrinology* 147 (2006): 5740–51.

Peplow, M. "Chernobyl's legacy." *Nature* 471 (2011): 562–65.

Rajkovic, V., M. Matavulj, and O. Johansson. "Studies on the synergistic effects of extremely low-frequency magnetic fields and the endocrine-disrupting compound atrazine on the thyroid gland." *Int. J. Radiat. Biol.* 86 (2010): 1050–60.

Relic, B., et al. "Genistein induces adipogenesis but inhibits leptin induction in human synovial fibroblasts." *Lab. Invest.* 89 (2009): 811–22.

Riu, A., et al. "Peroxysome proliferator-activated receptor γ is a target for halogenated analogues of bisphenol-A." *Environ. Health Perspect.*, 2011 May 11.

Rudel, R. A., et al. "Food packaging and bisphenol a and bis(2-ethyhexyl) phthalate exposure: findings from a dietary intervention." *Environ. Health Perspect.* 119 (2011): 914–20.

Sathyapalan, T., et al. "The effect of soy phytoestrogen supplementation on thyroid status and cardiovascular risk markers in patients with subclinical hypothyroidism: a randomized, double-blind, crossover study." *J. Clin. Endocrinol. Metab.* 96 (2011): 1442–49.

Sosić-Jurjević, B., et al. "Suppressive effects of genistein and daidzein on pituitary-thyroid axis in orchidectomized middle-aged rats." *Exp. Biol. Med.* (Maywood) 235 (2010): 590–98.

Stoewsand, G. S. "Bioactive organosulfur phytochemicals in Brassica oleracea vegetables—a review." *Food Chem. Toxicol.* 33 (1995): 537–43.

Tabb, M. M., and B. Blumberg. "New modes of action for endocrine-disrupting chemicals." *Mol. Endocrinol.* 20 (2006): 475–82.

Tadi, K. "3,3'-Diindolylmethane, a cruciferous vegetable derived synthetic anti-proliferative compound in thyroid disease." *Biochem. Biophys. Res. Commun.* 337 (2005): 1019–25.

Tanaka, T., et al. "Congener-specific polychlorinated biphenyls and the prevalence of diabetes in the Saku Control Obesity Program." *Endocr. J.*, 2011 May 7.

Tang-Péronard, J. L., et al. "Endocrine-disrupting chemicals and obesity development in humans: a review." *Obes. Rev.*, Apr 2011, doi:10.1111/j.1467-789X.2011.00871.x.

Verhoeven, D. T., et al. "Epidemiological studies on brassica vegetables and cancer risk." *Cancer Epidemiol. Biomarkers Prev.* 5 (1996): 733–48.

Walsh, B. "Flame retardants in everyday products may be a health hazard, scientists say." *Time*, October 28, 2010.

Watkins, D. J., et. al. "Exposure to PBDEs in the office environment: evaluating the relationship between dust, handwipes, and serum." *Environ. Health Perspect.*, 2011 Jun 30.

Yang, H. Y., J. R. Chen, and L. S. Chang. "Effects of soy protein hydrolysate on blood pressure and angiotensin-converting enzyme activity in rats with chronic renal failure." *Hypertens. Res.* 31 (2008): 957–63.

Zhou, Y., et al. "The effect of soy food intake on mineral status in premenopausal women." *J. Women's Health* (Larchmt.) 20 (2011): 771–80.

Chapter 9 Resources

Alberga, A. S., R. J. Sigal, and G. P. Kenny. "A review of resistance exercise training in obese adolescents." *Phys. Sportsmed.* 39 (2011): 50–63.

Anton, S. D., et al. "Effects of a weight loss plus exercise program on physical function in overweight, older women: a randomized controlled trial." *Clin. Interv. Aging* 6 (2011): 141–49.

Antunes-Correa, L. M., et al. "Exercise training improves neurovascular control and functional capacity in heart failure patients regardless of age." *Eur. J. Cardiovasc. Prev. Rehabil.*, 2011 Jun 22.

Astrup, A. "Thermogenesis in human brown adipose tissue and skeletal muscle induced by sympathomimetic stimulation." *Acta. Endocrinol. Suppl.* (Copenh.) 278 (1986): 1–32.

Ballard, T. P., et al. "Effect of resistance exercise, with or without carbohydrate supplementation, on plasma ghrelin concentrations and postexercise hunger and food intake." *Metabolism* 58 (2009): 1191–99.

Benov, L. "Comments on 'The effect of training type on oxidative DNA damage and antioxidant capacity during three-dimensional space exercise.'" *Med. Princ. Pract.* 20 (2011): 493–94.

Blundell, J. E., and N. A. King. "Effects of exercise on appetite control: loose coupling between energy expenditure and energy intake." *Int. J. Obes. Relat. Metab. Disord.* 22 (1998): S22–29.

Blundell, J. E., et al. "Cross talk between physical activity and appetite control: does physical activity stimulate appetite?" *Proc. Nutr. Soc.* 62 (2003): 651–61.

Broom, D. R., et al. "Influence of resistance and aerobic exercise on hunger, circulating levels of acylated ghrelin, and peptide YY in healthy males." *Am. J. Physiol. Regul. Integr. Comp. Physiol.* 296 (2009): R29–35.

Carey, D. G. "Quantifying differences in the 'fat burning' zone and the aerobic zone: implications for training." *J. Strength Cond. Res.* 23 (2009): 2090–95.

Carhuatanta, K. A., et al. "Voluntary exercise improves high-fat diet-induced leptin resistance independent of adiposity." *Endocrinology* 152 (2011): 2655–64.

CDC Exercise Guidelines, www.cdc.gov/physicalactivity/everyone/guidelines/index.html

Church, T. S., et al. "Trends over 5 decades in U.S. occupation-related physical activity and their associations with obesity." *PLoS One* 6 (2011): e19657.

De Souza, R. W., et al. "High-intensity resistance training with insufficient recovery time between bouts induce atrophy and alterations in myosin heavy chain content in rat skeletal muscle." *Anat. Rec.* (Hoboken), Jun 2011, doi:10.1002/ar.21428.

Demartini, J. K., et al. "Comparison of body cooling methods on physiological and perceptual measures of mildly hyperthermic athletes." *J. Strength Cond. Res.*, 2011 Jul 13.

Dimeo, F. C., et al. "Effect of aerobic exercise and relaxation training on fatigue and physical performance of cancer patients after surgery. A randomised controlled trial." *Supportive Care in Cancer* 12 (2004), doi:10.1007/s00520-004-0676-4.

Ding, Q., Z. Ying, and F. Gómez-Pinilla. "Exercise influences hippocampal plasticity by modulating brain-derived neurotrophic factor processing." *Neuroscience*, 2011 Jun 29.

Erdmann, J., et al. "Plasma ghrelin levels during exercise—effects of intensity and duration." *Regul. Pept.* 143 (2007): 127–35.

Feigenbaum, M. S., and M. L. Pollock. "Prescription of resistance training for health and disease." *Med. Sci. Sports Exerc.* 31 (1999): 38–45.

Folland, J. P., and A. G. Williams. "The adaptations to strength training: morphological and neurological contributions to increased strength." *Sports Med.* 37 (2007): 145–68.

Gabriel, D. A., G. Kamen, and G. Frost. "Neural adaptations to resistive exercise: mechanisms and recommendations for training practices." *Sports Med.* 36 (2006): 133–49.

Guerra, B., et al. "Is sprint exercise a leptin signaling mimetic in human skeletal muscle?" *J. Appl. Physiol.*, 2011 Jun 9.

Harrison, C. L., et al. "The impact of intensified exercise training on insulin resistance and fitness in overweight and obese women with and without polycystic ovary syndrome." *Clin. Endocrinol* (Oxf.), 2011 Jun 28, doi:10.1111/j.1365-2265.2011.04160.x.

Hopps, E., and G. Caimi. "Exercise in obesity management." *J. Sports Med. Phys. Fitness* 51 (2011): 275–82.

Hsu, Y. W., et al. "Aging effects on exercise-induced alternations in plasma acylated ghrelin and leptin in male rats." *Eur. J. Appl. Physiol.* 111 (2011): 809–17.

Ide, B. N., et. al. "Time course of strength and power recovery after resistance training with different movement velocities." *J. Strength Cond. Res.* 25 (2011): 2025–33.

Iwanaga, M., and M. Tsukamoto. "Preference for musical tempo involving systematic variations of presented tempi for known and unknown musical excerpts." *Percept. Mot. Skills* 86 (1998): 31–41.

Johnson, F., et al. "Could increased time spent in a thermal comfort zone contribute to population increases in obesity?" *Obes. Rev.* 12 (2011), doi:10.1111/j.1467-789X.2010.00851.x.

Karacabey, K. "The effect of exercise on leptin, insulin, cortisol and lipid profiles in obese children." *J. Int. Med. Res.* 37 (2009): 1472–78.

Karageorghis, C. I., et al. "Revisiting the relationship between exercise heart rate and music tempo preference." *Res. Q. Exerc. Sport.* 82 (2011): 274–84.

King, J. A., et al. "Differential acylated ghrelin, peptide YY3-36, appetite, and food intake responses to equivalent energy deficits created by exercise and food restriction." *J. Clin. Endocrinol. Metab.* 96 (2011): 1114–21.

King, N. A., V. J. Burley, and J. E. Blundell. "Exercise-induced suppression of appetite: effects on food intake and implications for energy balance." *Eur. J. Clin. Nutr.* 48 (1994): 715–24.

Klem, M. L., et al. "A descriptive study of individuals successful at long-term maintenance of substantial weight loss." *Am. J. Clin. Nutr.* (66) 1997: 239–46.

Konishi, I., et al. "Aerobic exercise improves insulin resistance and decreases body fat and serum levels of leptin in patients with hepatitis C virus." *Hepatol. Res.*, 2011 Jun 28, doi:10.1111/j.1872-034X.2011.00833.x.

Kozak, L. P., R. A. Koza, and R. Anunciado-Koza. "Brown fat thermogenesis and body weight regulation in mice: relevance to humans." *Int. J. Obes.* (Lond.) 34 (2010): S23–27.

Leah, E. "Metabolic disease: muscular fat burning." *Nat. Rev. Mol. Cell Biol.* 11 (2010): 314.

Li, J. B., et al. "Effects of exercise on the levels of peptide YY and ghrelin." *Exp. Clin. Endocrinol. Diabetes* 119 (2011): 163–66.

Libardi, C. A., et al. "Effect of resistance, endurance and concurrent training on TNF-α, IL-6 and CRP." *Med. Sci. Sports Exerc.*, 2011 Jun 21.

Ligibel, J. A., et al. "Impact of a mixed strength and endurance exercise intervention on levels of adiponectin, high molecular weight adiponectin and leptin in breast cancer survivors." *Cancer Causes Control* 20 (2009): 1523–28.

Lo, M. S., et al. "Training and detraining effects of the resistance vs. endurance program on body composition, body size, and physical performance in young men." *J. Strength Cond. Res.*, 2011 Jul 8.

Martins, C., et al. "Effects of exercise on gut peptides, energy intake and appetite." *J. Endocrinol.* 193 (2007): 251–58.

Marzullo, P., et al. "Acylated ghrelin decreases during acute exercise in the lean and obese state." *Clin. Endocrinol.* (Oxf.) 69 (2008): 970–71.

McGuire, M. T., et al. "What predicts weight regain among a group of successful weight losers?" *J. Consult. Clin. Psych.* 67 (1999): 177–85.

Miyazaki, S., et al. "Effect of exercise training on adipocyte-size-dependent expression of leptin and adiponectin." *Life Sci.* 86 (2010): 691–98.

Moran, L. J., et al. "Lifestyle changes in women with polycystic ovary syndrome." *Cochrane Database Syst. Rev.* 7 (2011): CD007506.

National Weight Control Registry Database, www.nwcr.ws/default.htm

Nieman, D. C., et al. "Upper respiratory tract infection is reduced in physically fit and active adults." *Br. J. Sports Med.*, 2010 Nov 1.

Parker-Pope, T. "Workplace cited as a new source of rise in obesity." *New York Times*, May 26, 2011.

Plante, T. G., et al. "Exercising with an iPod, friend, or neither: which is better for psychological benefits." *J. Health Behav.* 35 (2011): 199–208.

Plotnikoff, R. C., et al. "Predictors of physical activity in adults with type 2 diabetes." *Am. J. Health Behav.* 35 (2011): 359–70.

Poirier, P., and J. P. Després. "Exercise in weight management of obesity." *Cardiol. Clin.* 19 (2001): 459–70.

Ratey, J. J., and J. E. Loehr. "The positive impact of physical activity on cognition during adulthood: a review of underlying mechanisms, evidence and recommendations." *Rev. Neurosci.* 22 (2011): 171–85.

Ribeiro, M. O., et al. "Expression of uncoupling protein 1 in mouse brown adipose tissue is thyroid hormone receptor-beta isoform specific and required for adaptive thermogenesis." *Endocrinology* 151 (2010): 432–40.

Ropelle, E. R., et al. "IL-6 and IL-10 anti-inflammatory activity links exercise to hypothalamic insulin and leptin sensitivity through IKKbeta and ER stress inhibition." *PLoS Biol.* 8 (2010), pii:e1000465.

Safdar, A., et al. "Endurance exercise rescues progeroid aging and induces systemic mitochondrial rejuvenation in mtDNA mutator mice." *Proc. Natl. Acad. Sci. USA* 108 (2011): 4135–40.

Schneider, S., et al. "Exercise, music, and the brain: is there a central pattern generator?" *J. Sports Sci.* 28 (2010): 1337–43.

Shepstone, T. N., et al. "Short-term high- vs. low-velocity isokinetic lengthening training results in greater hypertrophy of the elbow flexors in young men." *J. Appl. Physiol.* 98 (2005): 1768–76.

Touvra, A. M. "Combined strength and aerobic training increases transforming growth factor-β1 in patients with type 2 diabetes." *Hormones* (Athens) 10 (2011): 125–30.

van der Vlist, B., C. Bartneck, and S. Mäueler. "moBeat: Using interactive music to guide and motivate users during aerobic exercising." *Appl. Psychophysiol. Biofeedback* 36 (2011): 135–45.

Walsh, N. P., et al. "Position statement. Part one: immune function and exercise." *Exerc. Immunol. Rev.* 17 (2011): 6–63.

Watanabe, M., et al. "Cold-induced changes in gene expression in brown adipose tissue: implications for the activation of thermogenesis." *Biol. Pharm. Bull.* 31 (2008): 775–84.

Watanabe, M., et al. "Differential effects of cold exposure on gene expression profiles in white versus brown adipose tissue." *Appl. Biochem. Biotechnol.*, 2011 May 10.

Weil, R. "Burning fat through exercise." *Diabetes Self Manag.* 19 (2002): 85–86, 88, 90.

Wyatt, H. R., et al. "Lessons from patients who have successfully maintained weight loss." *Obesity Management* 1 (2005): 56–61.

Yamada, M., et al. "Effect of resistance training on physical performance and fear of falling in elderly with different levels of physical well-being." *Age Ageing*, 2011 Jul 4.

Yang, J., et al. "Functional evolution of leptin of ochotona curzoniae in adaptive thermogenesis driven by cold environmental stress." *PLoS One* 6 (2011): E19833.

Zelasko, C. J. "Exercise for weight loss: what are the facts?" *J. Am. Diet. Assoc.* 95 (1995): 1414–17.

Chapter 10 Resources

Agil, A., et al. "Beneficial effects of melatonin on obesity and lipid profile in young Zucker diabetic fatty rats." *J. Pineal. Res.* 50 (2011), doi:10.1111/j.1600-079X.2010.00830.x.

Aldabal, L., and A. S. Bahammam. "Metabolic, endocrine, and immune consequences of sleep deprivation." *Open Respir. Med. J.* 5 (2011): 31–43.

Alvarez, G. G., and N. T. Ayas. "The impact of daily sleep duration on health: a review of the literature." *Prog. Cardiovasc. Nurs.* 19 (2004): 56–59.

Axelsson, J., et al. "Beauty sleep: experimental study on the perceived health and attractiveness of sleep deprived people." *BMJ* 341 (2010), doi:10.1136/bmj.c6614.

Ayala, G. X., et al. "Away-from-home food intake and risk for obesity: examining the influence of context." *Obesity* (Silver Spring) 16 (2008): 1002–08.

Baron, K. G., et al. "Role of sleep timing in caloric intake and BMI." *Obesity* (Silver Spring) 19 (2011), doi:10.1038/oby.2011.100.

Beaudoin, C. E., and T. Hong. "Health information seeking, diet and physical activity: an empirical assessment by medium and critical demographics." *Int. J. Med. Inform.* 80 (2011): 586–95.

Beccuti, G., and S. Pannain. "Sleep and obesity." *Curr. Opin. Clin. Nutr. Metab. Care* 14 (2011): 402–12.

Benedict, C., et al. "Acute sleep deprivation reduces energy expenditure in healthy men." *Am. J. Clin. Nutr.* 93 (2011): 1229–36.

Bertisch, S. M., C. C. Wee, and E. P. McCarthy. "Use of complementary and alternative therapies by overweight and obese adults." *Obesity* (Silver Spring) 16 (2008): 1610–15.

Birch, L. L., and K. K. Davison. "Family environmental factors influencing the developing behavioral controls of food intake and childhood overweight." *Pediatr. Clin. North Am.* 48 (2001): 893–907.

Borer, K. T., et al. "Appetite responds to changes in meal content, whereas ghrelin, leptin, and insulin track changes in energy availability." *J. Clin. Endocrinol. Metab.* 94 (2009): 2290–98.

Brainard, G. C., et al. "Sensitivity of the human circadian system to short-wavelength (420-nm) light." *J. Biol. Rhythms* 23 (2008): 379–86.

Brondel, L., et al. "Acute partial sleep deprivation increases food intake in healthy men." *Am. J. Clin. Nutr.* 91 (2010): 1550–59.

Buison, A., et al. "Augmenting leptin circadian rhythm following a weight reduction in diet-induced obese rats: short- and long-term effects." *Metabolism* 53 (2004): 782–89.

Canapari, C. A., et al. "Relationship between sleep apnea, fat distribution, and insulin resistance in obese children." *J. Clin. Sleep Med.* 7 (2011): 268–73.

Chan, J. C., and J. Sobal. "Family meals and body weight. Analysis of multiple family members in family units." *Appetite*, 2011 Jul 7.

Chaput, J. P., et al. "Longer sleep duration associates with lower adiposity gain in adult short sleepers." *Int. J. Obes.* (Lond.), 2011 Jun 7, doi:10.1038/ijo.2011.110.

Chaput, J. P., L. Klingenberg, and A. Sjödin. "Do all sedentary activities lead to weight gain: sleep does not." *Curr. Opin. Clin. Nutr. Metab. Care* 13 (2010): 601–07.

Christakis, N. A., and J. H. Fowler. "The spread of obesity in a large social network over 32 years." *New Eng. J. Med.* 357 (2007): 370–79.

Contreras-Alcantara, S., K. Baba, and G. Tosini. "Removal of melatonin receptor type 1 induces insulin resistance in the mouse." *Obesity* (Silver Spring) 18 (2010): 1861–63.

Cortés-Gallegos, V., et al. "Sleep deprivation reduces circulating androgens in healthy men." *Arch. Androl.* 10 (1983): 33–37.

Dalen, J., et al. "Pilot study: Mindful Eating and Living (MEAL): weight, eating behavior, and psychological outcomes associated with a mindfulness-based intervention for people with obesity." *Complement. Ther. Med.* 18 (2010): 260–64.

Dattilo, M., et al. "Sleep and muscle recovery: endocrinological and molecular basis for a new and promising hypothesis." *Med. Hypotheses*, 2011 May 6.

Dechamps, A., et al. "Pilot study of a 10-week multidisciplinary tai chi intervention in sedentary obese women." *Clin. J. Sport Med.* 19 (2009): 49–53.

Diéguez, C., et al. "New insights in ghrelin orexigenic effect." *Front. Horm. Res.* 38 (2010): 196–205.

Djuric, Z., et al. "A pilot trial of spirituality counseling for weight loss maintenance in African American breast cancer survivors." *J. Natl. Med. Assoc.* 101 (2009): 552–64.

Dyzma, M., et al. "Neuropeptide Y and sleep." *Sleep Med. Rev.* 14 (2010): 161–65.

Escobar, C., et al. "Scheduled meals and scheduled palatable snacks synchronize circadian rhythms: Consequences for ingestive behavior." *Physiol. Behav.* 104 (2011): 555–61.

Field, T. "Tai chi research review." *Complement. Ther. Clin. Pract.* 17 (2011): 141–46.

Garaulet, M., et al. "Ghrelin, sleep reduction and evening preference: relationships to CLOCK 3111 T/C SNP and weight loss." *PLoS One* 6 (2011): e17435.

Gupta, S. "Dear (food) diary. A new study shows that dieters can double their weight loss by jotting down what foods they eat." *Time*, August 4, 2008.

Hanifin, J. P., et al. "High-intensity red light suppresses melatonin." *Chronobiol Int.* 23 (2006): 251–68.

Harsch, I. A., et al. "Leptin and ghrelin levels in patients with obstructive sleep apnoea: effect of CPAP treatment." *Eur. Respir. J.* 22 (2003): 251–57.

Hayes, A. L., et al. "Sleep duration and circulating adipokine levels." *Sleep* 34 (2011): 147–52.

Hollis, J. F., et al. "Weight loss during the intensive intervention phase of the weight-loss maintenance trial." *Am. J. Prev. Med.* 35 (2008): 118–26.

Huang, W., et al. "Circadian rhythms, sleep, and metabolism." *J. Clin. Invest.* 121 (2011), doi:10.1172/JCI46043.

Ivanova, E. A., et al. "Altered metabolism in the melatonin-related receptor (GPR50) knockout mouse." *Am. J. Physiol. Endocrinol. Metab.* 294 (2008): e176–82.

Jin-Mei, L., and X. Yi. "Obesity and sleep-related breathing disorders." *Zhongguo Yi Xue Ke Xue Yuan Xue Bao* 33 (2011): 235–38.

Johns, M. W. "A new method for measuring daytime sleepiness: the Epworth sleepiness scale." *Sleep* 14 (1991): 540–45.

Karatsoreos, I. N., et al. "Disruption of circadian clocks has ramifications for metabolism, brain, and behavior." *Proc. Natl. Acad. Sci. USA* 108 (2011): 1657–62.

Kaufman, N. "Internet and information technology use in treatment of diabetes." *Int. J. Clin. Pract. Suppl.* (Feb 2010): 41–46.

Kim, J., et al. "Inflammatory pathways in children with insufficient or disordered sleep." *Respir. Physiol. Neurobiol.*, 2011 May 5.

Kluge, M., et al. "Effects of ghrelin on psychopathology, sleep and secretion of cortisol and growth hormone in patients with major depression." J. Psychiatr. Res. 45 (2011): 421–26.

Kluge, M., et al. "Ghrelin increases slow wave sleep and stage 2 sleep and decreases stage 1 sleep and REM sleep in elderly men but does not affect sleep in elderly women." *Psychoneuroendocrinology* 35 (2010): 297–304.

Kluge, M., et al. "Effects of ghrelin on psychopathology, sleep and secretion of cortisol and growth hormone in patients with major depression." *J. Psychiatr. Res.* 45 (2011): 421–26.

Knutson, K. L., et al. "The metabolic consequences of sleep deprivation." *Sleep Med. Rev.* 11 (2007): 163–78.

Knutson, K. L., and E. Van Cauter. "Associations between sleep loss and increased risk of obesity and diabetes." *Ann. NY Acad. Sci.* 1129 (2008): 287–304.

Knutson, K. L. "Sleep duration and cardiometabolic risk: a review of the epidemiologic evidence." *Best Pract. Res. Clin. Endocrinol. Metab.* 24 (2010): 731–43.

Kodama, S., et al. "Effect of web-based lifestyle modification on weight control: a meta-analysis." *Int. J. Obes.* (Lond.), 2011 Jun 21, doi:10.1038/ijo.2011.121.

Kong, A. P., et al. "Associations of sleep duration with obesity and serum lipid profile in children and adolescents." *Sleep Med.*, 2011 Jun 18.

Konturek, P. C., T. Brzozowski, and S. J. Konturek. "Gut clock: implication of circadian rhythms in the gastrointestinal tract." *J. Physiol. Pharmacol.* 62 (2011): 139–50.

Korkmaz, A., et al. "Role of melatonin in metabolic regulation." *Rev. Endocr. Metab. Disord.* 10 (2009): 261–70.

Leproult, R., and E. Van Cauter. "Effect of 1 week of sleep restriction on testosterone levels in young healthy men." *JAMA* 305 (2011): 2173–74.

Leproult, R., and E. Van Cauter. "Role of sleep and sleep loss in hormonal release and metabolism." *Endocr. Dev.* 17 (2010): 11–21.

Lira, F. S., et al. "Exercise training improves sleep pattern and metabolic profile in elderly people in a time-dependent manner." *Lipids Health Dis.* 10 (2011): 113.

MacLeod, M. "Restaurant industry opposes calorie content disclosure." *CMAJ* 183 (2011): 348–49.

Marc, I., et al. "Mind-body interventions during pregnancy for preventing or treating women's anxiety." *Cochrane Database Syst. Rev.* 7 (2011): CD007559.

Martins, P. J., et al. "Orexin activation precedes increased NPY expression, hyperphagia, and metabolic changes in response to sleep deprivation." *Am. J. Physiol. Endocrinol.* Metab. 298 (2010): E726–34.

McClafferty, H. H. "Integrative approach to obesity." *Pediatr. Clin. North Am.* 54 (2007): 969–81.

McIver, S., M. McGartland, and P. O'Halloran. "'Overeating is not about the food': women describe their experience of a yoga treatment program for binge eating." *Qual. Health Res.* 19 (2009) 1234–45.

Morselli, L., et al. "Role of sleep duration in the regulation of glucose metabolism and appetite." *Best Pract. Res. Clin. Endocrinol. Metab.* 24 (2010): 687–702.

Must, A., and S. M. Parisi. "Sedentary behavior and sleep: paradoxical effects in association with childhood obesity." *Int. J. Obes.* (Lond.) 33 (2009): S82–86.

Naska, A., et al. "Eating out, weight and weight gain. A cross-sectional and prospective analysis in the context of the EPIC-PANACEA study." *Int. J. Obes.* (Lond.) 35 (2011): 416–26.

Nayak, N. N., and K. Shankar. "Yoga: a therapeutic approach." *Phys. Med. Rehabil. Clin. N. Am.* 15 (2004): 783–98.

Nduhirabandi, F., et al. "Chronic melatonin consumption prevents obesity-related metabolic abnormalities and protects the heart against myocardial ischemia and reperfusion injury in a prediabetic model of diet-induced obesity." *J. Pineal. Res.* 50 (2011), doi:10.1111/j.1600-079X.2010.00826.x.

Nedeltcheva, A. V., et al. "Sleep curtailment is accompanied by increased intake of calories from snacks." *Am. J. Clin. Nutr.* 89 (2009): 126–33.

Obbagy, J. E., et al. "Chefs' opinions about reducing the calorie content of menu items in restaurants." *Obesity* (Silver Spring) 19 (2011): 332–37.

Pejovic, S., et al. "Leptin and hunger levels in young healthy adults after one night of sleep loss." *J. Sleep Res.* 19 (2010), doi:10.1111/j.1365-2869.2010.00844.x.

Piggins, H. D. "Human clock genes." *Ann. Med.* 34 (2002): 394–400.

Reiter, R. J., et al. "Obesity and metabolic syndrome: association with chronodisruption, sleep deprivation, and melatonin suppression." *Ann. Med.*, 2011 Jun 13.

Richards, C. A., and A. G. Rundle. "Business travel and self-rated health, obesity, and cardiovascular disease risk factors." *J. Occup. Environ. Med.* 53 (2011): 358–63.

Ríos-Lugo, M. J., et al. "Melatonin effect on plasma adiponectin, leptin, insulin, glucose, triglycerides and cholesterol in normal and high fat-fed rats." *J. Pineal. Res.* 49 (2010), doi:10.1111/j.1600-079X.2010.00798.x.

Riva, G., et al. "Interreality: the experiential use of technology in the treatment of obesity." *Clin. Pract. Epidemiol. Ment. Health* 7 (2011): 51–61.

Rosa Neto, J. C., et al. "Sleep deprivation affects inflammatory marker expression in adipose tissue." *Lipids Health Dis.* 9 (2010): 125.

Sahay, B. K. "Role of yoga in diabetes." *J. Assoc. Physicians India* 55 (2007): 121–26.

Schmid, S. M., et al. "Short-term sleep loss decreases physical activity under free-living conditions but does not increase food intake under time-deprived laboratory conditions in healthy men." *Am. J. Clin. Nutr.* 90 (2009): 1476–82.

Simpson, N. S., S. Banks, and D. F. Dinges. "Sleep restriction is associated with increased morning plasma leptin concentrations, especially in women." *Biol. Res. Nurs.* 12 (2010): 47–53.

Skene, D. J. "Optimization of light and melatonin to phase-shift human circadian rhythms." *J. Neuroendocrinol.* 15 (2003): 438–41.

Steiger, A., et al. "Effects of hormones on sleep." *Horm. Res.* 49 (1998): 125–30.

Steiger, A., et al. "Ghrelin in mental health, sleep, memory." *Mol. Cell Endocrinol.* 340 (2011): 88–96.

Steiger, A. "Sleep and the hypothalamo-pituitary-adrenocortical system." *Sleep Med. Rev.* 6 (2002): 125–38.

St-Onge, M. P., et al. "Short sleep duration increases energy intakes but does not change energy expenditure in normal-weight individuals." *Am. J. Clin. Nutr.*, 2011 Jun 29.

Tan, D. X., et al. "Significance and application of melatonin in the regulation of brown adipose tissue metabolism: relation to human obesity." Obes. Rev. 12 (2011), doi:10.1111/j.1467-789X.2010.00756.x.

Telles, S., et al. "Short term health impact of a yoga and diet change program on obesity." *Med. Sci. Monit.* 16 (2010): CR35–40.

Van Cauter, E., et al. "Impact of sleep and sleep loss on neuroendocrine and metabolic function." *Horm. Res.* 67 (2007): S2–9.

Van Cauter, E., and K. L. Knutson. "Sleep and the epidemic of obesity in children and adults." *Eur. J. Endocrinol.* 159 (2008): S59–66.

von Schantz, M. "Phenotypic effects of genetic variability in human clock genes on circadian and sleep parameters." *J. Genet.* 87 (2008): 513–19.

West, K. E., et al. "Blue light from light-emitting diodes elicits a dose-dependent suppression of melatonin in humans." *J. Appl. Physiol.* 110 (2011): 619–26.

Wing, R. R., and R. W. Jeffery. "Benefits of recruiting participants with friends and increasing social support for weight loss and maintenance." *J. Consult. Clin. Psychol.* 67 (1999): 132–38.

Zee, P. C., and C. A. Goldstein. "Treatment of shift work disorder and jet lag." *Curr. Treat. Options Neurol.* 12 (2010): 396–411.

Zirlik, S., et al. "Leptin, obestatin and apelin levels in patients with obstructive sleep apnoea syndrome." *Med. Sci. Monit.* 17 (2011): CR159-64.

Chapter 11 Resources

Adam, C. L., and J. G. Mercer. "Hypothalamic neuropeptide systems and anticipatory weight change in Siberian hamsters." *Physiol. Behav.* 74 (2001): 709–15.

Bacon, L., and J. Matz. "Intuitive eating: enjoy your food, respect your body." *Diabetes Self Manag.* 27 (2010): 44–5, 47–8, 51.

Cole, R. E., and T. Horacek. "Applying precede-proceed to develop an intuitive eating nondieting approach to weight management pilot program." *J. Nutr. Educ. Behav.* 41 (2009): 120–26.

Cole, R. E., and T. Horacek. "Effectiveness of the 'My Body Knows When' intuitive-eating pilot program." *Am. J. Health Behav.* 34 (2010): 286–97.

Dalen, J., et al. "Pilot study: Mindful Eating and Living (MEAL): weight, eating behavior, and psychological outcomes associated with a mindfulness-based intervention for people with obesity." *Complement. Ther. Med.* 18 (2010): 260–64.

Fasano-Ramos, M. "Mindful meals: a holistic approach to eating." *Beginnings* 24 (2004): 1.

Framson, C., et al. "Development and validation of the mindful eating questionnaire." *J. Am. Diet. Assoc.* 109 (2009): 1439–44.

Hammond, M. "Mindful eating. Tuning in to your food." *Diabetes Self Manag.* 24 (2007): 36, 38, 40.

Mathieu, J. "What should you know about mindful and intuitive eating?" *J. Am. Diet. Assoc.* 109 (2009): 1982–87.

Mayer, E. A. "Gut feelings: the emerging biology of gut-brain communication." *Nat. Rev. Neurosci.* 12 (2011), doi:10.1038/nrn3071.

Outland, L. "Intuitive eating: a holistic approach to weight control." *Holist. Nurs. Pract.* 24 (2010): 35–43.

Sharma, A. M., and R. Padwal. "Obesity is a sign—over-eating is a symptom: an aetiological framework for the assessment and management of obesity." *Obes. Rev.* 11 (2010): 362–70.

Stanton, R. A. "Nutrition problems in an obesogenic environment." *Med. J. Aust.* 184 (2006): 76–79.

Wansink, B. "From mindless eating to mindlessly eating better." *Physiol. Behav.* 100 (2010): 454–63.

Wansink, Brian. *Mindless Eating: Why We Eat More Than We Think*. New York: Bantam Dell, 2006.

BON! Acknowledgments

I would like to thank all my patients, past and present, for the knowledge they have given me about successful weight loss and the privilege of being involved in their care.

I want to thank Robyn Spizman, Neil Shulman, M.D., Randy Kessler, and Bobbie Christmas for their support, advice, and encouragement. I want to thank my agent, John Willig, for his incredible support and direction. I would also like to thank Jill Alexander and Will Kiester from Fair Winds Press, whose guidance and advice made this book possible. I want to thank Laura Smith for her brilliant editing of this manuscript. I would also like to thank my office staff, Janet Baldwin, R.N., Misty Roland, L.P.N., Fran Ritter, R.N., Deborah English, Annie Goode, Bethany Burton, and Shundalyn Vanderhorst. I would also like to give a special thanks to my officer manager, Bethany Knott, who has helped keep my office running smoothly while I took time off to write this book.

I want to thank my mother and father, Howard and Sheryle Isaacs. I would like to give an extra-special thanks to the two loves of my life, my wife, Fiona Isaacs, and my daughter, Arabella Isaacs. These two people gave me the love and support I needed to complete this project. Thank you for everything!

—Scott Isaacs, M.D.

About the Author

Scott Isaacs, M.D., F.A.C.P., F.A.C.E., is a board-certified endocrinologist in Atlanta, Georgia, and widely considered to be one of the leading weight-loss experts in the U.S.. Dr. Isaacs is a faculty member at Emory University School of Medicine and the medical director for Atlanta Endocrine Associates and their award-winning weight loss program.

Dr. Isaacs has been honored with numerous awards, including being listed in Castle Connolly Top Doctors for the past four years. His peers voted him Best Physician in *Lifestyles Magazine* in 2010 and 2011. The online *Citysearch Guide* announced Dr. Isaacs's weight loss program as its 2009 "Best of Citysearch" winner.

Author Jillian Michaels called Dr. Isaacs the "guru of all things hormonal" and referenced his books in her *New York Times* bestselling book, *Master Your Metabolism*. Dr. Isaacs has been profiled on CNNHealth.com, LIVESTRONG.com, WebMD.com, and many other websites. The American Association of Clinical Endocrinologists lists Dr. Isaacs's books as resources for practicing endocrinologists.

He has also been featured in national publications, including *Health, Ladies' Home Journal, Better Homes and Gardens, Fitness, Shape, Parents, Redbook, Family Circle, Men's Health, Better Health and Living, Good Housekeeping, Glamour, Chicago Tribune, The Atlanta Journal-Constitution, Atlanta, FirstHealth, Prevention, Women's World, First for Women* and others. Dr. Isaacs has provided expert commentary on radio and television news programs, including CNN Headline News, CNN Health, National Public Radio, and local NBC, ABC, CBS, and Fox news affiliates. He appeared as a weight-loss expert on TBS Superstation's *Movie and a Makeover*.

Dr. Isaacs is actively involved with the American Association of Clinical Endocrinologists at a national level, serving on several committees. He serves on the board of directors for the Atlanta chapter of the American Diabetes Association, as a Medical Advisor for Cushing's Help and Support Group, and is past president of the Georgia chapter of the American Association of Clinical Endocrinologists.

Dr. Isaacs attended Emory College and graduated magna cum laude and Phi Beta Kappa with a degree in psychology. Research from work in the Emory

Honors Program resulted in his first publication on hormones and the brain in 1991. He went on to Emory University School of Medicine, continuing for his residency in internal medicine and fellowship in endocrinology, lipids, diabetes, and metabolism, where he received a research grant from the National Institutes of Health and won an award from the American College of Physicians for published research on diabetes and obesity.

He has published clinical and basic science research on diabetes, obesity, and bone metabolism. His publications in peer-reviewed medical journals include the *Journal of Endocrinology and Metabolism, Diabetes Care, Journal of Cellular Physiology*, and the *Journal of Critical Care*. His articles have been referenced and cited in many subsequent publications, including a listing as a primary reference in the 2006 *American Association of Clinical Endocrinologists and American Diabetes Association Consensus Statement on Inpatient Diabetes and Glycemic Control.*

A frequent speaker to national and international groups, Dr. Isaacs is a diplomat of the American College of Physicians and a fellow of the American College of Physicians and the American College of Endocrinology.

Dr. Isaacs lives with his wife and five-year-old daughter in Atlanta, Georgia. He enjoys taking walks in Atlanta, hiking, swimming, fishing, cooking, and learning Spanish.

Visit www.IntelligentHealthCenter.com, www.BeatOvereatingNow.com, and www.YourEndocrinologist.com for more information about Dr. Isaacs.

Index